MW01140863

ROADMAP TO REMISSION

A Practical Guide to Hashimoto's Healing

MARC RYAN, L.AC.

Paperback ISBN: 978-1515022879

To the three most important & influential women in my life:

My partner, Olesia, my daughter, Ava,
and my mother, Joyce.

This book would not have been possible
without your love and support.

Table of Contents

For additional material cited in the book, visit the supplemental area on our website: www.hashimotos-diet.com/roadmap-to-remission-supplemental
Username: TenThousand Password: Roadmap1!

PREFACE

I wrote this book to help people suffering from the debilitating effects of Hashimoto's Thyroiditis. Therefore, I have set a personal goal to help 10,000 people and I hope that you will be one of those 10,000.

I sincerely hope that you will experience at least some small victories along your journey and then build on those victories to gain some positive healing momentum and, eventually, reach remission.

In my personal and clinical experience I have found that to achieve remission from Hashimoto's you must:

- First, understand, at least somewhat, what's happening to your body.

- Second, identify the problem areas and prioritize which are the worst.

- Third, acquire the necessary tools for fixing those problem areas and start initiating the healing process.

- And, lastly, follow through with the healing process on all systems of the body that have been impacted and use that healing to build positive momentum.

In addition, I sincerely hope to provide you with some inspiration of what is possible, some practical knowledge, and some clinical insights that you might not have had before about this incredibly complex, mysterious, and beautiful vessel we call the human body.

If you are like many of the people with Hashimoto's that I've worked with then you may be easily overwhelmed and have difficulty retaining a lot of information. We've tried to design the book to minimize that discomfort and to allow you easy access to the information.

As you read, you'll notice that the paragraphs are small, and headlines summarize the essential ideas and there are many summaries and recaps of important take-aways at the end of each chapter.

In addition, you may observe that the subject matter is not strictly technical and clinical in nature. In my opinion, real life is more than physiology and science.

And healing requires more than a laundry list of drugs and supplements. So this book includes plenty of emotion, stories, opinions, spirit, and curiosity.

And I'll warn you, I can be irreverent, opinionated, silly, and unorthodox. It's all in the name of trying to bring life to material that can sometimes be a bit dry and boring.

That's what makes things fun and worth pursuing. I'd be bored writing a book without that. And you'd probably be bored reading it. If you're looking for a standard grade medical text, this book is probably not for you.

Most importantly, keep in mind that remission is not the magical disappearance of your Hashimoto's. Nor is it a cure or license to go back to the things that made you sick in the first place.

Remission is a journey.

It involves taking responsibility for your life and circumstances and doing whatever is necessary to change that life and those circumstances.

The road to your remission should be ever evolving and growing, and it should be a process that you continue to improve upon and refine.

So it is not a destination. Getting there is just half the battle. Staying there is the other half. And the only way you can stay there is to be committed for the long haul.

Measurable goals should be:
- normal thyroid lab tests,
- antibodies within the normal range, and
- a healthy range for a number of other key indicators (which we will explore in upcoming chapters of the book).

These goals are just that. They are meant to be targets. You may not reach them 100%. And that's ok, not reaching them 100% does not mean you will have failed or that you should give up and quit trying. These are just numbers and numbers in isolation are never a complete measure of success or failure.

One important thing to remember about laboratory tests is that they are not meaningful outside the context of what you are experiencing in your own body.

So you must always be aware of what is happening in your body, of how you feel and also of what factors led up to that. Try to pay attention to both the good and the bad.

What you feel is clinically relevant and diagnostically important. And, really everything you do and try is just a test. What happens as a result is data that we can use; it provides us with clues and valuable information.

In addition, one should never keep forcing a solution when the evidence before you plainly shows you that it isn't working.

You must change your plan when that happens.

This can be tricky, but it is possible to do it if you have a system.

Unfortunately, this is usually not part of the mainstream approach. With conventional medicine, medication is often the first treatment option, diet and lifestyle changes are ignored or dismissed and the experiences that you have within your body are not given the importance that they deserve.

To address this problem and offer an alternative way of approaching healing that does take important factors like diet, lifestyle, physical, emotional and spiritual experiences into account, I've created a simple system for you to use.

The A.P.A.R.T. System

It's called **The A.P.A.R.T. System,** because this approach stands apart and so will your results if you use it.

This is a simple, easy-to-remember acronym for getting better results that aren't based on protocols, dogma, or preconceived ideas.

It goes like this:

A&A

T&T

P&P

R&R

A&A

The A.P.A.R.T. System

Each letter has two ideas that are associated with it.

1. A = Ask and Assess

Data has healing power, if you know what data to collect and analyze and you know what to do with that information. (Both are big "ifs.")

You need to ask what the symptoms are and assess the different systems of the body to find out where these symptoms are coming from.

And every bodily system and lifestyle practice needs to be a suspect. Don't exclude something because you're attached to it, feel like you can't do without it or have decided that it isn't a problem.

Everything in your life should be evaluated with equal scrutiny and if it isn't working to make you better, it may have to be eliminated.

This includes people, places, and things like your favorite foods and drinks.

2. P = Prioritize and Plan

Not everything has the same level of importance. This is what 80/20 teaches us (20 per cent of your issues cause 80 per cent of your symptoms – I've described in more detail in the Introduction).

Some things are having more of an impact than others. Figure out which they are (the positive feedback loops – or the things that are repeated and reinforced in your body and mind) and focus on those first, then make a plan to fix them.

I have created a Cheat Sheet in the back of the book that contains what I think are the most common 20 percent issues that cause 80 percent of our problems.

3. A = Act and Adapt

Act and put your plan into motion. Then observe what the results are. Double down on what works and change what doesn't. And results should be apparent relatively quickly. If they aren't, you need to make changes.

The common practice of a doctor or practitioner prescribing something and then telling the patient to come back in three to six months is not the best approach, in my opinion. That's way too long, especially if it isn't working.

4. R= Reassess and Readjust

Retest, reassess and ask all over again. Figure out what worked and what didn't. Double down on what worked and either eliminate or recreate a plan for what didn't.

It sounds obvious, but it is often overlooked or forgotten. Testing and reevaluating what you have done to see the result of your treatment is essential for good care.

Quick side note here: In my opinion, what I have learned over many years of practice is that you need to trust what the data is telling you. In most cases, when you make the right choice, you start feeling better.

Things like a "healing crisis," a "die off," or a "detox reaction" sometimes occur, but they can also be a cover for incompetence. The right decision should result in a positive result relatively quickly.

If you are doing something and you aren't getting better or you continue to feel worse, or it causes more discomfort, pain, and adverse symptoms, then you need to question whether that is the best course of action.

Eliminate it, reduce variables, and find out which part of what you are doing is causing that reaction or set of symptoms.

And all of this should not be done on the basis of lab tests alone. With Hashimoto's it must include a thorough examination of the signs and symptoms as well.

Remember, what you feel is diagnostically important and clinically relevant.

5. T = Try and Try Again

Keep doing it, keep refining, keep building on the positive results and keep looking for the remaining positive feedback loops that are causing vicious cycles.

People sometimes give up before giving a certain approach a chance. Or they get some good results and then slide back to their old ways of doing things. When you find something that works, keep doing it. Don't quit and don't give up.

> *Our main goal is the transformation of vicious cycles into positive healing momentum. This means you start to feel better and then you build on that success.*

Lab work and symptoms should all confirm that this has taken place.

Again, lab tests must always be viewed in context to how you feel. It is the combination of these two factors that determine success or failure.

In addition, you must create realistic goals that are small enough to achieve and then build upon them. Acknowledge and celebrate your small victories. You can't go from sick to perfect in a couple of weeks.

As I said, remission is a journey. It is measured by how you feel, by your lab tests and by your quality of life.

In other words, this journey is all about creating a lifestyle that will sustain and foster ongoing success.

INTRODUCTION

Over the last 2 years I've had over 2,000 conversations with people who suffer with this disease. And one of the most common questions I am asked is, "Why doesn't my doctor understand what is happening with Hashimoto's?"

People often share with me that they feel like they're being dismissed and that they're symptoms are not being taken seriously by their doctors.

They want to know "Why do doctors say things like, 'Hashimoto's isn't a real disease' or 'People just want to blame everything on this disease.'"

I don't know exact reasons or circumstances, but one possible explanation is the popularity of the drug, Synthroid. This drug is a synthetic form of the thyroid hormone, T4.

It is also the number one branded synthetic hormone therapy for thyroid disease and the most widely prescribed medication in the United States.

According to Drugs.com, total sales of Synthroid in 2013 exceeded $800 million.

Because of the drug's popularity and market share, the manufacturers have influenced the research and treatment of hypothyroidism and Hashimoto's.

And, of course, doctors know how important thyroid hormone is in the body, so there are good reasons for prescribing this drug. But, there are also consequences to the dogma of this approach.

Dogma is a principle or set of principles laid down by an authority, in this case, the medical establishment, as incontrovertibly true. In other words, don't argue with me, this is the truth. Period, end of conversation.

The problem is that these principles aren't always true when you're dealing with autoimmune diseases, like Hashimoto's. And when this treatment doesn't work, it can have a big impact on people's lives.

Two Theories that Lead to Declines in Quality of Life

As a result; the following two theories have become common practice:

#1: Synthetic T4 has been deemed the only treatment that is necessary and it is the standard of care for the majority of patients with Hashimoto's and hypothyroidism.

Results are considered confirmed by testing TSH (Thyroid Stimulating Hormone) and total T4.

As long as TSH is within the normal range, the patient is considered healthy.

For all intents and purposes, this practice is nothing more than TSH management with synthetic T4.

#2: The thyroid can be lost and simply replaced by thyroid hormone medication. Letting the thyroid be destroyed by autoimmunity or having it surgically removed are both presented as viable, and sometimes preferred, treatment options.

This may seem like an exaggeration, but I have heard from many patients that this was the advice that they received from their physicians. And they were told that supplementation with synthetic T4 would be all that is necessary once the thyroid is removed or destroyed.

This is supported by research, as well. Ho TW et al, in a study published in 2011 in the American Journal of Surgery, found that the percentage of patients having total thyroidectomy increased from 17.6% (from 1993-1997) to 39.4% (from 2003-2007) for benign, non-cancerous, thyroid disease.

Both of these theories have widespread consequences that affect the lives of millions worldwide, and sometimes dramatically. And the problem is that this approach doesn't always work and often doesn't address the underlying cause (the autoimmune process).

To date, I have yet to find a single evidence based study that supports the idea that removing the target tissue (that part of the body being attacked) removes autoimmunity from the body.

Furthermore, that theory makes no sense physiologically. The more we learn about autoimmunity, the more we understand it to be systemic and it often attacks multiple body parts.

These two theories are also responsible for the decline in quality of life for some people, which can mean loss of employment due to inability to work and function. In addition, it may also result in painful alienation and isolation from friends, family, and loved ones.

This is not a quality of life that any sane person would feel is acceptable or desirable. Yet, this is often the accepted quality of care in today's conventional medical system.

When these two approaches don't work, patients are then sometimes advised to get psychiatric evaluations and prescribed anti-depressants and anti-anxiety medications.

It doesn't have to be this way. There are other options for approaching this problem.

In upcoming chapters we will explore alternatives to this methodology and seek to understand, first, what is happening in the bodies of people who suffer from Hashimoto's. And, second, we will examine the solutions that are effective for treating this disease.

Beforehand, I'd like to share my own personal story so that you can get a sense of where I'm coming from and why I'm so passionate about the work that I do.

My Story

I have Hashimoto's, one of my children has Hashimoto's and my entire practice is devoted to studying, researching, treating, and helping people recover from this disease.

I'm also a graduate of Cornell University and a licensed acupuncturist and herbalist who practices functional medicine. If you don't know what this means, it is a marriage of Western diagnostic testing and natural medicine.

I've been in practice about thirteen years. My life isn't perfect, but I have an amazing life today. I'm able to be present for my family, spend time with my kids, and walk my crazy dog twice a day.

I have the energy to do all this and to work with lots of people with Hashimoto's. I'm excited about jumping out of bed in the morning.

Treating Hashimoto's Is All I Do

I love what I do, and all I do is treat Hashimoto's. It's all I want to do. And there's no end to the challenges, believe me!

My passion has enabled me to work with people all over the world. I am fortunate to have the clinical and personal experience to really help my Hashimoto's patients—something that mainstream medicine, as we have seen, sometimes struggles to do.

But I didn't really plan it this way. I didn't wake up one day and decide to become "The Hashimoto's Guy." There was a time when I was suffering from the debilitating effects of this disease just like many other people.

I was tired all the time, I couldn't sleep, I was in pain, I couldn't concentrate, my memory was shot, I couldn't focus, my digestion was horrible, my joints hurt, I had gained about 20 pounds of bloating and inflammation, and the worst thing was I had this really bad eye pain that just wouldn't stop.

Finally, I went to a couple of eye doctors, and one of them did a battery of tests. At that point they discovered that I had a marker called HLA-B27, which is seen in people with Crohn's disease, and something called ankylosing spondylitis, which can cause the vertebrae in your spine to fuse.

I had some chronic back pain, but I didn't really have any other symptoms. Doctors told me that we'd wait and see and when it got bad enough, they'd put me on immunosuppressant therapy and pain relieving drugs to completely disable my immune system and, hopefully, keep me out of pain.

As a functional medicine practitioner, that made no sense to me. Wait until my spine is severely damaged and then do something to disable another part of my body?

The truth is, if a person has to live through that, it evolves into a gradual, or sometimes not so gradual, loss of function and quality of life. It's miserable. I've worked with people who had gotten to that point.

I'm Not Going that Route

Well... no! No, no. I didn't want to go that route.

In response, I started treating myself using what I knew from functional medicine. I began a strict autoimmune diet and took some supplements. Through that, I was able to start to get my life back.

Then, something interesting happened, I lost those extra 20 lbs. and because I could actually see my body differently, I discovered some nodules on my thyroid.

I went to see an MD friend, and he sent me for an ultrasound and some blood tests. Thank God, the nodules were not cancerous, but my antibodies were really high, and I was diagnosed with Hashimoto's.

And the funny thing was, I was in the same place all over again. My doctor said, "Yeah, you have elevated antibodies (at the time my TPO (Thyroid Peroxidase antibodies) was 1200), but all your thyroid numbers are in the normal range."

He continued, "So we're going to keep an eye on it and when it gets bad enough, we'll put you on Synthroid, and that will take care of it."

So, once again, do nothing until my thyroid is sufficiently destroyed and then act. It was then that the light went on in my head and I realized. . .

"There is nothing for us!"

Holy crap, I thought to myself, most emphatically, *there is nothing for those of us who are in this in between stage of discovering we have autoimmune disease and major destruction of the tissue that's being attacked. Nothing.*

This doctor was well intentioned; he was a personal friend. I know he had my best interest at heart. Yet, that was all he had to offer.

It was then that I decided to devote my life to finding other ways of solving this problem that could turn people's lives around ***before*** it was too late.

So I had to really step up what I was doing and had to study a lot to try and figure out how to heal this disease because I was determined not to let it ruin my life.

I started my website www.hashimotoshealing.com and our Facebook support group www.facebook.com/hashimotoshealing about two years ago so that I could share information and support my patients.

My hope was to reach a few hundred people and share some things that I had learned. Since then, this endeavor has absolutely exploded.

My site and others that are devoted to helping people heal from Hashimoto's and other autoimmune diseases have become popular, and I've come to realize that there are millions of people worldwide suffering from this disease.

Hashimoto's Is Everywhere

It's epidemic, and many are starting to take notice and are looking for alternatives to the treatment and care that is currently being offered. For a lot of us the current treatment approach is inadequate at best and just plain worthless at its worst.

Just to give you a sense of the sheer numbers, I have worked with more than 1,000 people with Hashimoto's in the last two years.

Here's what I've learned. The average age of people was 46, 96 % were female, 55 % were on thyroid hormone (the most common brand was Synthroid followed by Levothyroxine, Armour and Naturethroid), The most common symptoms were (in order) fatigue, brain fog, weight gain, depression, anxiety, hair loss/thinning, constipation and insomnia.

The majority of these conversations have been free consultations that I offer for two reasons: first, I genuinely want to help these people and, second, I want to learn everything I can. And what better way than to actually speak to the people who are living with Hashimoto's?

It's crazy. These are people who reached out to me who know they have this disease. Imagine how many more are out there who have not been diagnosed.

The majority of the people I've talked to, including myself, went a number of years before anyone figured out what was going on with them. Even though Hashimoto's is so widespread, it is commonly misdiagnosed or ignored.

So I really think we're seeing the tip of the iceberg.

My Mission in Life

Since this profound revelation, I have had the good fortune to study with some of the best teachers and practitioners in the world, like Dr. Datis Kharrazian, D.C..

I am indebted to him and many others (such as Matt van Benschotten, OMD, Dr. Sarah Ballantyne, PHD, Dr. Izabella Wentz, Chris Kresser, L.Ac., Mickey Trescott, Stacey Robbins, Dana Trentini and many more) who have devoted countless hours in study and research and have generously shared their knowledge, understanding, personal stories and experience with those of us who are hungry to find another way.

While it was not easy, I was gradually able to find my way. Today, I have plenty of energy, I have very little pain, I have figured out how to effectively treat and reverse the brain fog that really made it hard for me to function, and I have decided to commit my life to helping other people with Hashimoto's turn their lives around.

And it doesn't have to be so hard for you. Today, we are very fortunate to live in a time where there is a lot of great information at our disposal. The tricky part is sorting out which information is best for you and your unique set of circumstances.

The 80/20 Principle

I'd like to share something with you that's I think is a really valuable mindset for healing.

Earlier this year, I had an epiphany.

I stumbled upon something called the 80/20 principle.

It's an idea that is often applied to business. It's also called the Pareto Principle and, basically, it came from a discovery by an economist named Vilfredo Pareto.

Ok, so what does this have to do with Hashimoto's?

Well, it turns out that this basic idea applies to just about everything in the natural world.

Look around you...

...80 percent of the traffic travels on 20 percent of the roads in your town or city. Most people spend 80 percent of their time with 20 percent of their friends. Go look in your closet; you wear 80 percent of your clothes less than 20 percent of the time.

You can apply this to everything, including your body and your health. And it's not about the numbers.

The point is that there is an imbalance in cause and effect. Relatively few things cause the majority of results.

Why does this matter?

Well with Hashimoto's, if this is true, it means that 80 percent of our problems are caused by 20 percent of the things we need to work on.

Or let me put it another way:

If you are like many of the people that I have worked with, then 80 percent of your symptoms are caused by 20 percent of the choices you made today...

...now imagine if you could fix 80 percent of your symptoms fast by figuring out what those 20 percent choices are and then make some changes, making that 20 percent really count

This would then get you feeling 80 percent BETTER.

How awesome would that be:

To have 80 percent MORE ENERGY?

To have 80 percent more MENTAL CLARITY AND FOCUS?

To feel 80 percent HAPPIER?

To lose 80 percent of THAT WEIGHT YOU WANT TO LOSE?

To FEEL LIKE YOUR OLD SELF 80 percent of the time?

Who doesn't want that?

So, obviously, the most important thing is to figure out what is that 20 percent. Right?

After working with hundreds of people and studying thousands of hours and reading tons of research, I think I have a general sense of what this 20 percent encompasses for most people. This book will help you discover where it is for you.

One thing you can be sure of is that it is usually found in the things you spend the most time doing.

If we break that down to practical terms, that comes down to four areas of your life:

1. **Your DIET**

2. **How you handle STRESS AND BLOOD SUGAR—these are totally interrelated**

3. **EXERCISE—hugely important for your brain, for your immune system, for dealing with stress, etc.**

4. **And really getting good at FINDING THE 20% in your body.**

Get to know your body so you can identify where the problems are. Be conscious of what's happening on a daily basis, learn to take responsibility for the way your actions and behavior affect your health. It's remarkable how easy it is to forget that the answer is often inside of us.

And when you do become conscious, present and aware, it can dramatically improve your chances of getting better. Championships don't happen by accident. They are the result of a huge number of small conscious decisions.

Become a superstar in healing yourself. It is time, energy and effort that is well spent. In fact, I'll go out on a limb and say there is no better use of your time, energy and effort. When you lose your health, you often lose many of the things that make life worth living.

Understanding What Is Happening In Your Body

Metal

Fire

Earth

Five Elements of
Thyroid Health

Wood

Water

*All of the drawings in this book were illustrated by my son, Maklin Ryan.
These are really works of art! Thank you Maklin*

Chapter One

Functional Medicine &
The Five Elements of Thyroid Health

Western medicine seeks to determine what is going on with the body and how disease affects function, but is more focused on naming and identifying that disease. Pharmaceutical treatment often alters or shuts down some physiological process, working against nature and causing long-term unintended consequences. Then, over time, more drugs are added to shutdown or alter more functions.

Functional medicine, on the other hand, seeks to understand how disease affects the body's physiology. When things go wrong and people become sick, it is caused by something in their body not working properly. The treatment of Functional Medicine aims to correct what is going wrong and tries to help return the body to its normal function. The goal is to work with the body to help it heal itself.

Traditional Chinese Medicine (TCM) is, in many ways, the original functional medicine. Ancient Chinese doctors sought to figure out which parts of the body were not working properly and then tried to find ways to restore the body to balance.

TCM is, in my opinion, the original functional medicine. (Note: If you would like to learn more about the history of TCM, check out this article I wrote for Pubmed in the supplemental section for this book I have created on our website: https://hashimotos-diet.com/roadmap-to-remission-supplemental/)

TCM theory is designed to explain patterns of dysfunction and it has created systems that describe the relationships between the different parts of the body.

Two popular systems for explaining the relationships of different parts of the body are yin and yang and the 5 elements.

Yin and Yang Theory

Chinese Medical theory, though scientific in its own right, is built on a foundation of ancient philosophical thought. Many of these ideas are based on observations of the natural world and are the reason why TCM has remained a truly holistic approach to health and well being.

The Theory of Yin and Yang is one such philosophy. It is said to date back nearly 6,000 years to the third or fourth millennium B.C. and is attributed to an enlightened philosopher named Fu Shi (also credited with creating the I-Ching or Book of Changes).

The basic premise of yin and yang is the idea that the only constant factor in natural events is universal change.

In other words, nothing remains the same; no disease, no condition, no emotion, no treatment or diagnosis, absolutely everything is in a constant state of flux and, therefore, subject to the laws of change.

Yin and Yang Are Metaphors for Constant Change

Yin and Yang are metaphorical images used to express these constantly changing interactions. They have no fixed, precise definition.

Instead, they describe two broad categories of complementary concepts, which include the relationships of positive and negative, dynamic and inert, creative and destructive, gross and subtle, and kinetic and potential.

This is quite similar to the notion of dialectics as expressed in Western philosophy. Within dialectics, the whole is the sum of its parts and, in turn, part of the sum of a greater whole.

As these various components interact, they become their opposites, e.g., variables become constants, causes become effects, and the process of creation leads to destruction.

Furthermore, this idea is demonstrated in modern physics where sub-atomic interactions are the result of ever shifting polarities and constantly vacillating magnetic attractions and repulsions.

The Whole Universe Can Be Seen as Yin and Yang

The entire universe may be seen as the interplay and alternation of yin and yang.

Originally the Chinese characters for yin represented the moon, and yang represented the sun.

Gradually these terms were broadened to include yin as night and yang as day, yin as winter and yang as summer, and yin as female and yang as male.

In fact, there is nothing that cannot be viewed from the standpoint of yin and yang.

Examples of Yin

Yin is that which maintains and endures; it is nourishing and supports growth and development as well as being something that contracts and moves inward. Representing yin are:

- Earth
- Autumn
- Cold, coldness
- Moisture

Examples of Yang

Yang is that which is creative and generating; it develops and expands, and it is dynamic and full of movement. Representing Yang are:

- Heaven
- Spring, summer
- Heat, warmth
- Dryness

21

It is important to remember that yin and yang are not static concepts and that they are constantly influencing and determining one another. There is always some measure of yin within yang and vice versa.

In this fluid model it must be understood that neither yin nor yang can ever exist without the other.

In fact, extreme yin will become yang, an example of this can been seen in the popular expression, "the darkest hour is right before the dawn."

Naturally, the opposite is also true.

Yin and Yang In the Body

These yin and yang types of relationships become significant when they impact the body's anatomy and physiology, and it is precisely these designations that are used in the diagnosis of imbalances in TCM.

For a TCM practitioner, the name of the disease is of secondary importance. The primary key to the proper diagnosis of syndromes is the identification of the condition in terms of yin or yang.

Even Life is Yin and Yang

In order to understand what this means, let us examine these concepts in the context of human life.

Beginning at conception, the sperm, which is yang, unites with the yin ovum, and a new life is formed. As that life develops and progresses, the energetic stages of youth are yang; whereas the later years are yin as life slows and becomes more deliberate.

Each stage is also relative to the others and contains a measure of both yin and yang. For example, the quick growth of early childhood is yang within yang and the transition from middle age to old age is yin within yang.

Yin and Yang Anatomy & Physiology

We can also see this philosophy expressed in the human body. In respiration, the expansion of inhalation is yang, while the emptiness, which results from exhalation, is yin.

In digestion, the yin substance of food is transformed by the metabolic activity of yang. The yin blood carries the yang hormones, which cause many physiological changes.

The physical body itself expresses this model. The lower part of the body, which connects to the earth is yin, while the upper body and extremities are yang and free to move. The front, which can easily be protected is yin, while the exposed back is yang.

The internal organs, which are enclosed and protected, are yin relative to the surface of skin and muscle, which are yang.

In addition, the internal organs can be further differentiated into *fu* (yang), which are the "hollow" organs that are involved with digestion and elimination, and *zang* (yin) which are involved in assimilation and storage.

Each yin organ has a corresponding yang partner, which it is paired with and while these connections are not recognized in Western medical terms, they are often utilized in the treatment of disease in TCM.

Yin and Yang In Disease

Finally, disease and disease progression can be viewed using this paradigm. If the body's yang (the immune system) is weak, it will be unable to ward off the invasion of a pathogen.

If the yin is weak, there will not be enough nourishment and support for the yang and the result will be the same.

Expressed in other terms, without the substance the active immune system is weakened, and without activity the substance becomes vulnerable.

Therefore, if yin is deficient over time, then yang also becomes deficient and vice versa. Not only do yin and yang balance each other, they mutually generate one another.

It is precisely this balance that the TCM practitioner restores using various treatment strategies. The idea is to reestablish the body's innate ability to maintain health and defend itself from disease.

The nature and progression of disease can also be understood using this pattern. When a disease develops rapidly, it is in the acute or yang stage.

As it progresses and becomes more chronic, it enters the yin stage. Usually acute diseases affect the surface or superficial aspects of the body, while chronic diseases have already overwhelmed the body's defenses and gone deeper into the interior.

Hashimoto's is a perfect example. As it progresses, it travels deeper into the body and impacts more and more systems.

When conflicting signs are present, they usually point to a more complex condition, and the TCM practitioner must evaluate all the symptoms together to determine the appropriate treatment strategy.

Yin and Yang Summary

In summary, yin and yang are universal and extend into every aspect of life.

Because of its universal nature, this theory is a very useful tool for understanding natural phenomena and therefore can be a helpful diagnostic aid.

While this is an ancient paradigm, it is not primitive and though simple, it can be developed into surprising complexity.

5 Element Theory

Another theory that is used to understand relationships in the body is the 5 Element Theory. The 5 Elements really are a way of organizing functional relationships within the body.

The 5 Elements are earth, metal, water, wood, and fire and in the upcoming chapters, I will introduce them and go into more depth about each one.

Each 5 Element pairing has a yin and yang organ, a sphere of influence, and specific relationships to other elements in the system.

For example, the wood element involves the liver and gall bladder. Its sphere of influence includes the nervous system, the eyes, and tendons. Anger and depression are the negative emotions of the liver.

In regard to physiological function, all of these connections to the wood element can be explained. For example the liver and gall bladder work together to metabolize fat and fat-soluble toxins.

Many studies have shown that poor detoxification in the liver can lead to neurological disorders, chemical sensitivities, adverse drug reactions, fatigue, autoimmune disease, poor conversion of thyroid hormones, and so forth.

Serotonin is also synthesized in the liver, which can explain anger and depression as being emotions of the liver.

In addition, the liver element (wood) has a unique relationship with the spleen (earth element). The physiological functions that are described as belonging to the spleen include many of the functions of the pancreas.

If you look at it in this light, then many of the problems described as liver/spleen dysfunction, such as sugar balance and fat storage in the liver, start to make a whole lot of sense.

And you can see this repeated over and over again in the 5 Element relationships.

The fire element is the heart and small intestine.

What unites them? The cardiovascular system. Where is the highest concentration of fine capillaries in the body? They surround the small intestines.

The fire element has a unique relationship with the water element of the kidneys. Here we can see the role of the kidneys in managing blood pressure and its impact on the cardiovascular system.

Using 5 Element Theory to Explain Hashimoto's

To help my own understanding and to help explain the impact of hypothyroidism and Hashimoto's on the human body, I use the 5 Element System to describe how this disease impacts the whole body.

And because TCM doesn't do a great job explaining endocrine or neurological function, my approach is really a hybrid of both TCM and functional medicine filtered through my mind from many years of clinical experience.

I don't care about being a purist, I'm looking for answers.

What really matters is can this information and ways of looking at the body help us get better?

I believe the answer is **yes**, so let's jump in and explore this way of looking at the mind, body, and spirit effects of Hashimoto's Thyroiditis.

Chapter Two

Thyroid: Understanding the Terrain

One thing I want to do is to give you a good sense of what is happening in your body so that when you have a blood test or when you have symptoms, you can start to understand it and not feel like you are at the mercy of someone else to explain what is going on.

*The truth is, many medical providers have only a vague idea of what is really happening in **your** body.*

*The person who has the best understanding of that is **you**.*

In this and every chapter following, we are going to look at this disease from two perspectives: the Western medical model and the TCM model.

I have decided to do this because, in my view, Hashimoto's and any other "disease" for that matter, is really a mind, body, and spirit condition.

And if we are really interested in healing, which I believe we all are, then we need to understand that these things are all connected. And these connections extend everywhere in our bodies.

As we go through the anatomy and the physiology, I want you to keep in mind a couple of key ideas. First, the body is not a machine with isolated parts that you can replace like a car.

The body, like our world, is a series of interconnected ecosystems that are all living and breathing, and what happens in one eco-system influences and has consequences in others.

Ecosystems both inside and outside the body are connected

For example, if you dump a bunch of chemicals in the Mississippi river in Iowa, it's going to have an impact off the coast of Louisiana.

The same thing happens in your body every day. What you eat, the chemicals you are exposed to, the medications you take, they all have an impact.

Even a small amount of some things can have a pretty large impact on the body, such as environmental toxins, certain foods like gluten, and so forth.

The second thing to understand is that the body has a natural tendency to balance itself. This is called "homeostasis", and it is a very important process because a lot of what we are about to look at is the direct result of this very delicate balancing act.

A lot of symptoms from Hashimoto's are a result of this balancing act gone haywire. The hormones, the immune system, the digestive system, and the liver, etc.; somewhere, things have gotten all confused.

In this confusion normal function starts to go wrong. And this is the problem when trying to heal and treat Hashimoto's. So many connections cause many systems to get out of whack.

And that's the final point I want to make. Hashimoto's is complicated; it involves multiple systems.

It's not just a thyroid problem, or even a thyroid and immune system problem. It's a multi-system problem.

The best way to fix that type of problem is to make sure you keep the big picture in mind and don't get too fixated on one system alone.

You're the Single Parent of a Large Dysfunctional Family

The best analogy I have been able to come up with for describing Hashimoto's is that it is like being the single parent of a large dysfunctional family.

You're a single parent because, in most cases, you are on your own. The current Western medical approach to Hashimoto's treatment and management is failing. That's the simple truth.

So you are the parent, and your dysfunctional children are all the systems of your body that are being affected: the thyroid, the adrenals, the stomach, the kidneys, the liver, the gall bladder, the small intestines, the pancreas, the heart, the brain and more.

Every one of these systems can become compromised and then can affect all the other systems, just as one sibling affects all the others in a family.

And, if you think about it this way, then how do we heal a dysfunctional family?

Well, not by focusing treatment on only one child. **To heal the family you must treat the whole family, not just one or two children.**

That being said, let's take a look at the child that usually gets the most attention, first. The thyroid.

What Does the Thyroid Do?

Simple answer? **Everything!**

It is responsible for growth, for cell differentiation (helping cells grow into different specialists), reproduction, sex and intelligence, and brain development. It is responsible for pretty much everything.

Thyroid function also affects every major system of the body. Its influence is literally felt everywhere.

And through lots of signals coming from all over the body, a part of the brain called the hypothalamus gets messages that say, "Hey, we need more thyroid, hit the gas."

Or "Whoa! Slow our roll. We're getting too hyped up, less thyroid." This process happens all the time, 24/7, for your whole life.

And this is part of normal life. When you're cold, the hypothalamus sends a signal to speed things up to increase circulation so you get warmer. When you are stressed and freaking out, it sends signals to slow things down, so you can relax.

It sends nine different hormones to the pituitary. The thyroid is only one of nine systems that it is regulating.

The hypothalamus sends messages to the pituitary to release TSH

The hypothalamus sends these signals to the pituitary in the form of Thyroid Releasing Hormone. The pituitary is considered the master endocrine gland. The pituitary then releases TSH (Thyroid Stimulating Hormone) to the thyroid.

TSH is the test that many doctors believe is the only important test. The pituitary produces TSH.

Think about that for a second.

The most important test that determines your entire care (in some cases) is measuring something not coming from the thyroid. TSH is coming from your pituitary. And TSH is really a measure of pituitary function in relation to the thyroid and signals from the body.

Let me repeat that.

The most important test that determines your entire care (in some cases) is measuring something not coming from the thyroid. TSH is really a measure of pituitary function in relation to the thyroid and signals from the body.

So what happens next?

TSH stimulates TPO (Thyroid Peroxidase). With Hashimoto's one of the antibody tests performed is for TPO antibodies. Results can mean that your immune system is attacking this enzyme and destroying it.

TSH causes TPO (thyroid peroxidase) to create
T4 and T3 hormones in the thyroid using iodine

What TPO does is use iodine to create thyroid hormones T4 and T3. The majority of thyroid hormone produced is T4, about 93 percent, and the remaining 7 percent is T3. So when the immune system destroys enough of it, your thyroid produces too little thyroid hormone.

As we have already discussed, the most common drug that is prescribed for people with Hashimoto's, and for those who are hypothyroid, is Synthroid® or levothyroxine. This is synthetic T4. The rationale is that T4 is most of what your body produces, so that's all you need.

Well, the body doesn't really use T4. It has to be converted into something else that the body can use to get important stuff done like growing and making different cells, making babies, thinking, and learning. Super important stuff!

Where is T4 converted? Sixty percent is converted in the liver to T3, which is what the body uses.

60% of T4 is converted to T3 in the liver.
20% or more becomes reverse T3 (rT3)

The liver is a really important place for thyroid hormones to be made usable. This means that if the liver is congested or not working properly, then it will have trouble making thyroid hormone work. And if the gall bladder is not functioning properly, this can have a negative effect on this process as well.

And guess what? With Hashimoto's the liver is often not working properly for a bunch of reasons.

In the chapter on the Wood Element we will get into this in a lot more detail. Right now, it's big picture. The liver is really important for making thyroid hormone work.

From the liver, about 20 percent of this converted T3 becomes reverse T3, which the body can't use, but which can be a really useful test result because it tells us important information about how your body is using thyroid hormone.

Your body may actually push more T4 into reverse T3 when it wants to slow things down. Usually this occurs during times of extreme stress or when you have experienced physical trauma. But this can also happen gradually when you live your life in chronic stress mode.

20% is converted to active T3 in the digestive tract by good bacteria

Ok, next, 20 percent more of T4 is converted in the intestines. And the important thing there is your good bacteria. Remember the ecosystem?

Well, if you've taken lots of antibiotics or your diet is mostly processed and fast foods, or if you're taking lots of antacids or NSAIDS (like ibuprofen or acetaminophen), then your intestinal ecosystem might be totally out of whack.

This can have a big effect on whether or not you are able to convert and use thyroid hormone.

The Liver is very important for thyroid hormone conversion.

The ecosystem of the intestines is also very important for absorbing thyroid hormone.

The rest of T4 is converted in the peripheral tissues like the heart,
fat (adipose) and skeletal muscles

The last bits of T4 are converted in the tissues of the body: in the heart, in fat, in the glial cells of the brain, and in skeletal muscles. If you have inflammation in your body and autoimmune disease is, at its root, a disease of inflammation, then this will make converting thyroid hormone in your tissues more difficult.

Guess how many people with Hashimoto's have inflammation all over their bodies? Almost everyone. Take a look at this classic before and after thyroid photo.

Same woman in both photos.
Photo on the left, inflammation is plain to see

So can you see how these systems—the liver, the intestines, the tissues of your body are connected? They are all responsible for making thyroid hormone work. Problems in those places mean your medication may not be working that well at all.

This is one of the reasons why some people in the thyroid/Hashimoto's community advocate adding T3 to your medication regimen. You can take this in a synthetic form such as Cytomel® (liothyronine sodium) or you can get it with natural desiccated hormones like WP Thyroid®, Nature-Throid®, or Armour Thyroid.

And this does really help some people; but, again, nothing is perfect. There are so many variables here that you can still run into problems when taking natural desiccated hormones or adding T3.

For example, you may have an immune reaction to natural desiccated hormone, and too much T3 can make you really anxious, make you feel hyperthyroid symptoms, and it can have a powerful effect on heart muscle function.

What is best thing to do? Assess what is going on in your body and work on the other systems to improve conversion and absorption. **The importance of doing both can't be overstated.**

So, let's go back to the pituitary for a second. Remember how I said it was doing nine different jobs at once?

The pituitary doesn't really have time to focus only on the thyroid. It's like, "Hey, thyroid, you good? Cool! I got other stuff to do." Just like a mother with nine children, she only has so much time.

So one important question is, how does the pituitary absorb thyroid hormone? Because it is making TSH, and TSH is the be-all and end-all of treatment. Well, it turns out that the pituitary absorbs thyroid hormone a lot differently than the rest of the cells in your body.

Perhaps because of all of the demands on it, the pituitary is much more sensitive to thyroid hormone. It can sense it easily, whereas other cells in your body have to work a lot harder to get thyroid hormone into them.

This is important, clinically, because it is one of the reasons why you can have all normal lab numbers but feel like crap, especially if the doctor is only testing TSH.

Functional Hypothyroidism

One final thing I'd like to mention is a concept that is so common it is almost a cliché. And that is the idea of "functional hypothyroidism."

As I mentioned, I have worked with over 1,000 people with Hashimoto's, and by far the most common complaint and source of frustration is that they have normal lab tests but they still have all the classic hypothyroid symptoms.

They are tired all the time, they have terrible brain fog and memory issues, they're losing their hair, they're constipated, they have terrible digestive issues, they may have trouble losing weight, they're in pain, all those symptoms and more. You name it; they have all the classic symptoms.

Yet, their blood work is normal. So their doctors says, "You're fine, change your diet, get some exercise. I'll see you in 6 months."

The problem is, they aren't fine. And the reason is simple. Parts of their body (like their pituitary and their blood) are getting enough thyroid hormone. But it's not getting absorbed and it's not getting utilized.

There are many potential reasons for this but the important thing to understand is that, for all intents and purposes, they are hypothyroid and their health is declining as if they weren't getting enough thyroid hormone.

The reality is that they must be treated as though they are hypothyroid, and the process of conversion and absorption has to be improved.

Important Takeaway

So, what is the important take away here?

How you feel really matters when it comes to thyroid symptoms. It's not in your head. And your symptoms are very important when it comes to Hashimoto's because they are telling you whether your body is able to convert, absorb and utilize thyroid hormone.

Summary: Four Common Mistakes Doctors and Health Care Practitioners Make

Okay, so let's summarize the four common mistakes that doctors and health care practitioners make regarding the thyroid.

Mistake #1: They only test TSH. TSH is really more a measure of the pituitary's function with regard to the thyroid. While this is certainly an important test, it does not indicate actual thyroid hormone levels in the body.

And because the pituitary absorbs thyroid hormone differently than other cells in the body, TSH can be normal, but you can still feel lousy and be functionally hypothyroid.

Mistake #2: They ignore your symptoms. Sometimes doctors will say, "All your numbers are normal; you're doing great!" But you don't feel that way. With thyroid issues and Hashimoto's, in particular, what you feel is diagnostic and important. Do not let anyone tell you otherwise.

Mistake #3: They ignore other systems of the body and the thyroid's impact on those symptoms. Many symptoms can be related to poor thyroid function, low levels of thyroid hormone in your cells, or poor conversion and poor absorption of thyroid hormone by your cells.

It's important to pay attention to these other symptoms and to see the relationships of the thyroid with different parts of the body.

This observation matters because, in a number of instances, a problem in one place can create a vicious cycle of problems in both places.

For example, low thyroid function can cause the gall bladder to slow down and not do its job properly. This can cause toxins and hormones to build up in the liver making it unable to convert thyroid hormone properly. And on and on it goes.

Mistake #4: They think supplementing T4 is the only thing that matters. For some people, adding T3 to the mix can really help. But this approach alone ignores all the other important issues. Improving conversion, reducing inflammation, and making sure the other systems are functioning properly are all still necessary because this is much more than just a thyroid problem.

CASE STUDY

I'd like to tell you a story about how I helped a woman who struggled with Hashimoto's for forty-five years and had lost all hope find a way out to life that inspires everyone she knows.

This story is a perfect real life illustration of what we have just described and how things can be done differently. The wrong approach was used for many years, but once a changed to the right approach, amazing things happened.

Here's how it went down (used with permission).

She is a sixty-four-year-old woman who was diagnosed forty-five years ago (at age 18) with Hashimoto's.

She came to us after literally losing all hope after she had struggled for so long and just didn't believe it was possible to get better.

One night she was surfing the Internet and discovered our website and started reading, and it made sense to her.

She felt a small glimmer that maybe, just maybe, this time it would be different than the hundreds of other times she had tried and failed.

Like many people with Hashimoto's, she suffered from many digestive issues, bloating, gas, constipation, and a lot of reactions to many different foods.

She also experienced some fatigue after meals and felt irritable and shaky if meals were missed. She had undergone antibiotic treatment for two years for an infection that would not resolve.

In addition, she had heartburn and discomfort following her meals and she had to use antacids. She had a history of gall bladder issues and had her gall bladder removed several years before.

She had trouble sleeping, was under high amounts of stress, and didn't feel rested from sleep.

She was taking thyroid replacement hormone but had every hypothyroid symptom that you can think of: fatigue, cold hands and feet, brain fog and memory issues, weight gain, thinning dry hair, and she needed a lot of sleep to function.

What we saw in her were numerous vicious cycles at work, compounding symptoms and causing a downward spiral effect.

This is a perfect example of how Hashimoto's is a multi-system disorder and how other systems become impacted and lead to more hypothyroidism. This is what we call "functional hypothyroidism."

She was taking thyroid hormone; there was enough in her system, but it was not working.

She had also tried various combinations over the years including adding additional T3, and this made her feel horrible.

So, we set out to first find these various issues and then work on those systems and start to heal them.

With this approach, we can transform negative vicious cycles into positive healing momentum.

We found ample evidence of leaky gut and there were other digestive complaints. Getting her off of gluten, dairy, and soy had immediate benefits.

We went a step further and got her on a special diet designed to reduce systemic inflammation and to heal her gut. While we did that, we worked to support her liver and liver detoxification.

Her stomach acid symptoms went down dramatically with this approach, and we supplemented her to help increase stomach acid production, which eliminated many of the problems she was having.

This was also a great time to work on repairing the ecosystem of her gut that had been so disrupted by all the antibiotics.

In addition, we worked to balance blood sugar because cortisol is released when blood sugar drops, and she was just draining her adrenals and thyroid and then binging on sugar to try and get enough energy to get through the day.

Cortisol and systemic inflammation caused by sugar is a major factor in blocking thyroid hormone conversion and absorption.

This whole process took several months and we are happy to report that she now has an entirely new life today.

Here's an excerpt from an email she sent us:

"What a fabulous program....I just love it! It is the first time in my life that I have really invested the time and energy in taking care of ME!!!!

...I love my new life! I even purchased a bicycle! I hadn't ridden a bike for about thirty-plus years! Having a blast with it. Everything is more fun, and I feel like I have a new lease on life."

Diana D.
Washington

I spoke with Diana recently and what she shared with me literally had me in tears. Her enthusiasm and sense of gratitude made me feel like I was a Debbie Downer.

I'm serious!

I'm not claiming that everyone gets these results, nor is this something that just happened miraculously over night.

It took persistent hard work and it took looking in other parts of the body other than the thyroid.

She also continues to have some work to do. Something that's been progressing for forty-five years doesn't just disappear.

But she also deserves the credit for sticking to this and doing the hard work that resulted in such progress. That is something to celebrate!

What happened here is that we were able to create positive healing momentum and we were able to stop all these vicious cycles from continuing to make everything else worse.

That's key.

Vicious cycles are the result of positive feedback in the body.

Positive feedback is the result of repeated reinforcement.

And with Hashimoto's it can give you some pretty negative outcomes.

But when you work on them and reverse that negative momentum, you make the positive feedback work for you and you get healing momentum.

Does that make sense? This process involves working with nature and your body's natural tendencies.

HASHIMOMENT:
IS IT GOOD OR BAD?

I created Hashimoments for our Facebook support group. These are positive affirmations for people with Hashimoto's.

This one tells a story that really illustrates how we sometimes don't really know if something is good or bad.

It takes place in ancient China.

There was a wise farmer who, like so many farmers, toiled day in and day out in his village, doing all the work that needed to be done to run his farm and sustain his family.

Well, one day, one of his horses ran away. And his neighbor, who was a bit of a busy body, noticed.

He ran over and said, "Oh, I'm so sorry! That's such a tragedy. That's the horse you use for plowing and work. Oh this is bad!"

The farmer just shrugged and asked, "Is it?"

The very next day the horse returned with five wild horses running after him, and the farmer and his son were able to capture all of them.

His one old horse had become six!

The neighbor saw this and he ran over and said, "Oh my goodness! What good fortune, you are so lucky! Your one horse is now six. That's so great!"

The farmer just shrugged and asked, "Is it?"

The next day the farmer's son set to work on breaking in the new wild horses so that they could become work horses and be sold. As he was trying to ride one of them, he was thrown to the ground violently and landed badly and broke his leg.

The neighbor heard about this and ran over. He said, "Oh, I'm so sorry. What bad luck! Now your son can't work, and you're stuck with all these wild horses. Oh, this is bad!"

The farmer just shrugged once again and asked, "Is it?"

Two weeks later the army came to town.

They were requiring all young men in good health and of fighting age to go to the front and to join the Emperor's army in defending China from the invading Mongol hordes.

Many would die. But because the farmer's son had just broken his leg, he was spared and not drafted. They just took two of his new horses.

So you see, the moral of the story is that you never know what a given set of circumstances or a certain turn of events can mean.

When I was diagnosed with Hashimoto's, I thought my life was over. And for all intents and purposes, it was.

But that has turned out to be an incredible blessing because the life I am leading now is a new simpler and far more rewarding life.

And it was that adversity and difficulty I went through that got me to where I am today.

So don't be so quick to judge your circumstances. It may turn out to be a really good thing for you in the long run.

Chapter Three

The Chinese Medicine View of the Thyroid

Ok, now, let's look now at a different side—the energetic and emotional side of thyroid health. This really isn't strictly science, but parts of real life are more than science, physiology, and lab test results.

Looking at Hashimoto's and the thyroid from this perspective gives us clues about how we can understand what we are going through and how we can heal.

In TCM, the endocrine system is thought to come from the yang energy of the kidneys. In an energetic way, the kidneys are responsible for our individual power, or will.

The yang energy is the way the ancient Chinese understood hormones. And there is something to learn in their take on this. (For a review of yin and yang philosophy see chapter one.)

The ancient Chinese believed that we have all been given a certain reserve or fund of this yang energy at birth, and throughout our lives we use it. Sometimes we use it well and sometimes we use it foolishly. There are whole practices devoted to helping people use this reserve in a better way.

I studied with a Taoist master many years ago in New York City. His name is Mantak Chia. I remember going to his apartment in Chinatown and learning a special Tai Chi form he had adapted for small apartments. You can basically do the form right where you are standing.

One of things he did when I worked with him was to project energy into my eyeballs with his thumb. That was really intense and gave me a blast of yang energy! The reason he did this was to quickly fill up my reserves.

Here is a drawing that illustrates a Taoist practice called the Microcosmic orbit that I learned from Mantak Chia. It depicts an entirely different viewpoint.

Here we can see the process of transforming yang energy into other types of energy. For example, the ancient Taoists believed we could transform sexual energy into spiritual energy. They also believed this energy could be used to heal the internal organs and balance the nervous system.

Throughout history, Taoism has had a profound influence on Chinese medicine, and a number of Taoist ideas and practices are reflected in it.

The microcosmic orbit.
Energy circulates up the spine and down the front of the body.

I ask that you be open minded because some of this material is a bit "out there." But it also offers major insight into the emotional and spiritual aspects of the Hashimoto's journey.

Life Is A Journey

In my opinion, life itself is a journey. We are here together taking this journey regardless of our religious beliefs. And we are all having mind, body, and spirit experiences on a daily basis.

To this point we've already established that we aren't just lab test results, and that what we feel and experience does matter.

So let's look at this from a real experiential point of view and assume that we are part of this living universe that is made of an infinite amount of ecosystems.

Let's retrace the path we took previously and look at these processes from a Chinese medical/Taoist point of view.

First, the hypothalamus released what? TRH. And sent it where? To the pituitary.

The hypothalamus is a really magical place for Taoists. It represents an "on" switch to the Universal Force…. The force is strong Luke Skywalker…when your spirit awakens. This is where it is thought to happen.

This is also what connects us to the larger universe—the big dipper constellation, which contains the North Star, and has a special meaning in Taoist cosmology. And this is where we can connect to it. (We are not alone!)

The Pituitary is an Important Energy Center

Second, the pituitary is an important energy center. It is where yang energy is thought to be transformed to spiritual energy. When opened, the pituitary is a place of wisdom and direction.

When it is open, you have a strong sense of purpose and a direct and simple knowing. When it is closed, you may be indecisive; your mind may wander, and be directionless.

Meditation can really benefit the pituitary. It can create that balanced

The pituitary is where yang energy is transformed into spiritual energy

sense of purpose.

With Hashimoto's, hypothyroidism and inflammation of the brain can create some real cognitive problems. This happens because these processes can hamper neurotransmitter production and cause the immune cells of the brain to react and this can cause inflammation all over your brain (more on this in an upcoming chapter about the brain). Well, all of that affects the pituitary.

As we have seen, the pituitary sends information to the thyroid. The thyroid is considered an important energy center too. It is the place where communication and dreams are generated.

Of course, this is where your voice comes from, both physically and emotionally. When this center is open, your expression flows and you have greater lucidity in dreams. When it is closed, you may feel choked up and unwilling to change.

Third, we looked at how important the liver is for converting and transforming thyroid hormone. The liver is important for so many processes.

The sense organ connected to the liver is the eyes in Chinese medicine. Eye issues are a big part of thyroid problems! Both Graves disease and Hashimoto's have their own category of eye issues!

We can use the eyes in meditation practice to calm the nervous system and to send energy inward in what is a practice called the inner smile, where you smile into your organs and systems of your body and direct healing energy.

In terms of energy and emotion, the nature of the liver is kindness, which is maintained by the calmness and integrity of the heart. When the liver is out of balance, the negative emotion is anger, or anger turned inward—depression.

It is interesting to note that one of the most common next steps for physicians treating Hashimoto's patients is a referral for a psychological evaluation or simply prescribing anti-depressant medication.

When treatment with T4 doesn't result in the patient feeling better, then this is sometimes the next logical step.

You see? These ancient masters really understood this stuff on a deep level.

Finally, we went to the digestive tract. This is thought to be controlled by the spleen in Chinese medicine (although the intestines also belong to other organ systems).

In Chinese medicine, Hashimoto's treatments often address the spleen and kidneys because the yang energy is thought to be depleted and weak.

When your spleen is weak, you worry and obsess about things a lot. When it is healthy, you have a quality of fairness. You can see the big picture and be open.

The life issues of those of us with problems involving this yang energy revolve around the general theme of utilizing our resources appropriately.

Hashimoto's Can Be Seen as a Deficiency of Yang

Hashimoto's involves a deficiency of yang. We see this in various endocrine glands: the adrenals, the pancreas, the thyroid, and the pituitary.

Chinese treatment for hypothyroidism and Hashimoto's uses therapies that tonify or strengthen yang. It also addresses two other issues: what they call liver depression—interesting in light of what we saw about the liver and spleen deficiency, and digestive and blood sugar issues. (we will explore this in more detail in the chapters on the Earth and Wood Elements)

With acupuncture treatment we treat this energy by using points like Stomach 36 (located on the lateral part of the leg just below the kneecap) and the Japanese point LI 10 ½ (located on the , both important tonification and energy generating points.

Liver acupuncture points are really helpful for anger and depression. I always recommend trying a course of acupuncture before going on antidepressants, especially for mild to moderate depression.

The Ren and Du channels go up the back and center of the torso.

On the back, points for hypothyroidism often involve treating this energy pathway. The microcosmic orbit works with the energy of two main meridians, the Ren and Du channels. These run down the center of the front of the body and up the spine on the back.

These are our most primal channels and are thought to be formed at fertilization when the first cell is formed. These channels tap into the autonomic nervous system that is so overtaxed in our society and culture.

Treating the middle of the back area and back of the neck can also be very beneficial with Hashimoto's. Points in these areas have a potent effect on calming and balancing the thyroid.

In tandem with what you learned earlier, let's now look at some Hashimoto's and thyroid issues from a more energetic, emotional/spiritual perspective.

Wisdom is a Yang Virtue

Wisdom is the virtue associated with the yang energy of the kidneys, it empowers us to be in contact with our destiny from birth to death. This energy of the kidneys teaches us to use our wisdom to utilize the resources we have by listening to our inner voice rather than reacting to our fears.

Fear can make you impulsive and make you burn up your reserves. Engaging in meditation and prayer are good tools to develop that wisdom, and they enable you to get in touch with your inner voice so that you can use your energy in a more sustainable way.

You must learn to be like a boxer going twelve rounds. You always need to keep some energy in reserve, but you also need to go with the flow of the fight and use some of that energy at key times. Remain unattached to the outcome of the fight and focus instead on cultivating wisdom by listening to your inner voice.

That's an important part of this journey for treating Hashimoto's. We have to learn not to overdo it.

Recap

In the last chapter, we looked at the thyroid and how it works in your body.

We also looked at four common mistakes that many practitioners and doctors make. And we learned how what you are feeling really matters because it can absolutely be important diagnostically. In addition, we learned:

1. A number of spiritual and emotional pieces are attached to this entire process. Being connected to the universe, your higher power, however you want to look at it, is traditionally related to the hypothalamus.

2. The pituitary is a place of spiritual transformation—a place to find wisdom and direction and one of the parts of the body that really benefits from meditation practices. Meditation can benefit the thyroid as well.

3. The thyroid is a center for communication and dreams. Journaling your dreams and keeping track of them can be a way to tap into this energy.

4. The liver is, again, hugely important. It is connected to your eyes, to emotions of anger and depression (which can be anger turned inward).

5. The yang of the spleen and kidney is the energetic root of the endocrine system. This energy is responsible for many processes in the body, but has within it the seed of spiritual growth and development.

I don't know about you, but I find this of looking at the body to be inspiring. I like it because I believe we're more than just science and physiology. It's also interesting to think about spirit, energy and emotion, as well. Because therein lie the seeds of healing.

Chapter Four

Understanding Common Thyroid Tests

To this point, we've touched on some of the physiology and some of the spiritual and emotional aspects of Hashimoto's Thyroiditis.

We also looked at the more esoteric energetic side of things and looked at the life challenges that might be part of this whole journey we are going through.

That being said, I'm reminded of how important it is to **keep a journal.**

Make a habit of paying attention to what is going on with your body, mind, and spirit. Keep track of your symptoms and keep track of the foods you eat and other things that you interact with for clues on what might make things better or worse. This is valuable data.

In this chapter I want to get to some practical stuff and look more closely at what are the important thyroid tests to order and why.

Thyroid Testing

TSH—The Standard That No One Can Agree On

Thyroid stimulating hormone (TSH), also called thyrotropin, is released by the pituitary gland after the hypothalamus releases TRH (thyrotropin releasing hormone). TSH is the most common marker used to assess thyroid function.

Many laboratories have undertaken doing a test called a "thyroid cascade" in order to save themselves and insurance companies money.

Basically, if the TSH is deemed to be in the normal range, they will not order any other tests. This saves money because they aren't paying for additional testing, but it doesn't always serve people who are trying to get better.

The problem is, there isn't a lot of agreement about what the "normal range" is.

Since 2003, the American Association of Clinical Endocrinologists has recommended that the normal range run from 0.3 to 3.0, versus the older range of 0.5 to 5.5. So, according to the new standards, levels above 3.0 are evidence of possible hypothyroidism, and levels below 0.3 are evidence of possible hyperthyroidism.

However, there is disagreement among doctors, and some follow the older range, while others use the newer range.

TSH Is an Inverse Marker

An important thing to understand about TSH is that it is an inverse number when thinking about thyroid function. The higher it is, the more sluggish, and, generally, slow or hypoactive your thyroid is. The lower TSH is, the more high energy, fast and, generally, hyperactive your thyroid is.

Put another way: High TSH = hypothyroid, Low TSH = hyperthyroid.

TSH levels increase as T4 levels drop and TSH levels decrease as T4 levels rise. The reason this is the most popular test in today's medical model is because the only treatment offered for thyroid dysfunction is thyroid hormone replacement (usually in the form of synthetic T4) and that's what doctors are checking when they test your TSH.

A TSH test alone doesn't give you information about thyroid–pituitary communication, about T4 to T3 conversion in other parts of the body, or about whether your immune system is attacking your thyroid.

One important thing for Hashimoto's people to understand is that some antibodies can inhibit thyroid function by turning off, instead of stimulating, TSH receptors on cells. In this case, you will see high TSH and high antibodies.

Bottom Line on TSH

Laboratory range is somewhere between 0.3 to 3.0 and 0.5 to 5.5. That is a huge range and borders on the ridiculous. The lab range values are made based on the general population that goes to the·lab.

Most people who go to the lab are taking thyroid hormones, are poorly managed, or are completely undiagnosed (or all of the above), so this is not really a good measure of optimal thyroid health. Practitioners of functional medicine (like yours truly) look at a narrower range that we, and some endocrinologists, believe is a much better range for assessing a healthy thyroid.

This range is: 1.8 to 3.0. Notice it is higher on the low end and equal to or lower on the high end. Other people believe the "Goldilocks Zone," where it's just right, is somewhere between .5 and 2.0.

Regardless of the range, it is important to understand that these numbers mean nothing in isolation. They must be viewed in the context of your signs and symptoms, i.e., how you feel. You have to find your own ideal zone where you feel your best.

T4

The T4 test measures both bound and unbound thyroxine levels and is not a good marker for T4 activity when measured alone. Total T4 is increased with lower TSH and is decreased with higher TSH. It is decreased with low TSH when the pituitary gland is not functioning properly (pituitary hypofunction).

This begs the question: Are we measuring the pituitary or the thyroid?

Let's Look at Some Research

Well, there was an interesting study in *The Journal of Clinical Endocrinology & Metabolism* 2005; 90(12):6403–6409, titled <u>Thyroid Hormone Concentrations, Disease, Physical Function and Mortality in Elderly Men.</u>

This study of 403 men investigated the association between TSH, T4, free T4, T3, TBG, and reverse T3 (rT3) as well as parameters of physical functioning.

This study showed that TSH and/or T4 levels are poor indicators of tissue thyroid levels and, thus, in a large percentage of patients, cannot be used to determine whether a person is euthyroid (normal thyroid levels) at the tissue level.

In fact, T4 levels had a negative correlation with tissue thyroid levels (higher T4 levels were associated with decreased peripheral conversion of T4, low T3 levels, and high rT3).

Additionally, this study shows that rT3 inversely correlates with physical performance scores and that the T3/rT3 ratio is currently the best indicator of tissue levels of thyroid.

In addition, this study showed that increased T4 and rT3 levels and decreased T3 levels are associated with hypothyroidism at the tissue level with diminished physical functioning and the presence of a catabolic state (breakdown of the body).

Here's what this means:

- T4 is not a good test of thyroid hormone levels in the tissues of your body (where you need it to work). T3/rT3 ratio is a much better way to determine how much thyroid hormone is getting absorbed.

- Also, the combination of increased T4 and rT3 with decreased T3 levels meant that these people felt worse physically.

- This is the state of "functional hypothyroidism," that I described earlier. This is also important for figuring out if you are "functionally hypothyroid."

Another interesting point from the study was that many chronic diseases can lead to further decline in tissue sensitivity to hormones, diseases like diabetes, heart disease, hypertension, systemic inflammation, asthma, Chronic Fatigue Syndrome, fibromyalgia, rheumatoid arthritis, lupus, insulin resistance, obesity, chronic stress, and almost any other systemic illness.

What does that mean?

All of the issues just mentioned can be viewed as health issues that compromise energy (yang) in the body and cause systemic inflammation. These chronic conditions actually make conversion and tissue sensitivity worse.

Hashimoto's is also a systemic disease, and it often involves more than one of those other issues I just mentioned, making it the perfect recipe for "functional hypothyroidism".

Quick Recap: What tests did this study show were most helpful for figuring out if thyroid hormone is getting into the tissues/cells of the body?

T3, Reverse T3, and the T3/rT3 ratio.

Let's take a look at these tests.

T3: Total Triiodothyronine (TT3)

Total T3 gives you the total concentration of T3 in the blood. It is the preferred test for thyrotoxicosis (hyperthyroid condition like Graves disease).

Total T3 can also be useful for identifying T4 to T3 conversion problems in body tissue involving the enzyme 5'-deodinase.

This enzyme both converts T4 to T3 and stops T4 from working in the body.

Reverse T3

This test measures the amount of reverse T3 that is produced (You probably figured that out). Reverse T3 is usually created when there is an extreme amount of stress, for example, a serious car accident, or surgery, pregnancy, or really bad chronic stress.

It's no surprise that Reverse T3 is elevated after a stress response or after the body produces high amounts of the stress hormone cortisol.

Your body, especially the liver, is constantly converting T4 to rT3 as a way to get rid of any excess or unnecessary T4. As much as 40 percent of T4 goes to T3 and 20 percent of T4 goes to Reverse T3 any given day.

But in any situation where your body needs to conserve energy and focus on something else, such as dealing with Hashimoto's, it may increase the conversion of rT3, and then the T3 goes down, because there is less T4 to convert.

Examples are any kind of stress (especially extreme stress-like trauma, illness, terrible bosses), or being exposed to an extremely cold environment, diabetes, aging, or even being on certain drugs. But there's another reason for Hashimoto's folks.

We can get caught in a state of alarm, causing our body to increase rT3 in order to decrease the amount of T3 in our cells.

And the lower your T3, the worse you feel, including a lowered body temperature, fatigue, anxiety, weight gain, hair loss, pain and more...all common symptoms of Hashimoto's and hypothyroidism.

Sometimes your levels of rT3 can climb too high.

Why would you make too much rT3?

On top of the chronic stresses in your life are three common issues. The first two are related to your adrenals (low cortisol, high cortisol), and the third is related to your iron levels.

The adrenal issues can be divided into two categories:

1. When you have too much stress, your adrenal glands produce high amounts of cortisol to help you cope with ongoing hypothyroidism and lingering symptoms and conditions.

That alone is stressful. The extra cortisol inhibits the conversion of T4 to T3, and instead produces even larger amounts of rT3, creating an rT3 problem.

2. When that stress is ongoing, your adrenals will eventually become tired, dropping from high cortisol to a mix of high and low, or all low, and those low levels create adrenal fatigue, which can also cause problems.

We will explore this in more depth in the chapter on the Water Element.

When you don't make enough cortisol, thyroid hormones can build up in your blood. Your body responds by converting the T4 to excess rT3 because it has to do something with the extra T4.

The third issue involves iron deficiency anemia.

3. When iron levels or ferritin levels are low, as can be seen in your serum iron and saturation (quite common in thyroid patients), your red blood cells become less plentiful, and carrying thyroid hormones via your blood becomes inadequate, thyroid hormones can build up in your blood.

The body responds by producing excessive amounts of rT3 to clear out the excess T4.

You can have either an iron problem or a cortisol problem, or BOTH. Other health issues can cause you to have high rT3 as well, such as low B12, excess inflammation, and more. But the above are quite common and worthy of exploring first.

Another interesting thing to note is that interventions like meditation, qi gong, yoga and practices like them can be helpful in lowering reverse T3 levels. Don't always assume a drug or supplement is the only way to get better results.

Free T3 and Free T4

Other tests that are helpful are free T3 and free T4. These measure the free fractions of T3 and T4 or how much of T4 and T3 are available and active.

These are important because they are what the body uses. We want to know how much is available for the body to actually use.

The final thing to look at is the ratio of T3 or free T3 to reverse T3. It is generally accepted that this ratio should be 20 or more with T3 or 10 or more with free T3.

However, just like TSH, this number is just a number and means very little in isolation. You must also look at it in the context of how you feel and in the context of all the other numbers. This is the best way to figure out what it means. Again, trust how you feel.

Free T3 or T3/ rT3 Ratio

If free T3 or T3 is low and reverse T3 is high, then, as I stated above, you may have a state of "functional hypothyroidism." This means you aren't absorbing and/or converting well.

You might benefit from adding T3 to your medication, and you certainly need to address the underlying issues leading to poor conversion and utilization of hormones: things like stress, inflammation, liver, adrenals, and intestinal issues.

Calculating this result can be difficult if you are math challenged because different units are sometimes used for each test.

There's a great calculator for this at the Stop the Thyroid Madness website, http://www.stopthethyroidmadness.com/rt3-ratio/

Make sure you double-check that you are using the right units of measurement for each test when you use this calculator.

Thyroid Antibodies

When these antibodies are above the normal laboratory range, it can mean that your immune system is attacking your own tissue. When your body produces thyroid autoantibodies, it could create a hypo- or hyper- thyroid state.

These antibodies may also be elevated if there is thyroid cancer. Some antibodies can attach to TSH receptors, but they don't usually attack thyroid tissue, other parts of the immune system are responsible for this. We will explore this in more detail in upcoming chapters.

There are three autoantibodies that are tested. The first two are the most common:

1. **Thyroid Peroxidase Antibody (TPO Ab):** This antibody is the one that is usually high in autoimmune thyroid conditions like Hashimoto's. It is also known as microsomal antibody.

2. **Thyroglobulin Antibodies (TgAb):** These aren't seen high as often as TPO Ab. These antibodies are usually ordered when thyroid lab results seem strange because they can interfere with thyroid hormone production. TgAb is also used to monitor progress after surgery for removing the thyroid in thyroid cancer.

3. **Thyroid-Stimulating Hormone Receptor Antibody (TRAb or TSIAb):** This antibody is only ordered when a patient is hyperthyroid. Positive results usually mean Grave's disease.

Thyroid Ultrasound: Obviously, this isn't a blood test. It's an imaging test using ultrasound.

There are some people with Hashimoto's who may not have thyroid antibodies detectible in the blood. Having a thyroid ultrasound will help your physician determine the state of your thyroid and how badly it has been damaged in this process.

Chapter Five

Using the A.P.A.R.T. System to Heal the Thyroid

A&A

T&T

P&P

R&R

A&A

The A.P.A.R.T. System

As you may recall, the A.P.A.R.T system is a system I created to give you a template for fixing any imbalance or disorder in the body.

First, you must take inventory and figure out what the issues are. Then, your next step is to try various treatment approaches. After that you assess and take inventory again of what you did.

Figure out what worked and what didn't. And finally, over the long term, keep building on what works and keep eliminating what doesn't with the ultimate goal of reaching remission.

In this chapter we look at how you can apply this approach to the thyroid.

Make sure you get yourself a journal. Make a note of your symptoms and how you feel. Create a plan for dealing with these symptoms. Try some things. Record what the results were.

Double down on what worked, and change what didn't. Then, lather, rinse, repeat.

1. A = Ask & Assess

Ask: Do you have any of these hypothyroid and/or hyperthyroid symptoms?

Hypo: Tired/sluggish; Feel cold—hands, feet, all over; Require excessive amounts of sleep to function properly; Increase in weight even with low calorie diet; Gain weight easily; Difficult, infrequent bowel movements; Depression/lack of motivation; Morning headaches that wear off as the day progresses; Outer third of eyebrow thins; Thinning of hair on scalp, face, or genitals, or excessive hair loss; Dryness of skin and/or scalp; Mental sluggishness.

Do you have any of these hyperthyroid symptoms?

Hyper: Heart palpitations; Inward trembling; Increased pulse even at rest; Nervous and emotional; Insomnia; Night sweats; Difficulty gaining weight.

Assess: Test thyroid levels.

One note on testing: Two things to be aware of regarding testing are one, to order the right tests, and two, to know what to do with the data that the tests reveal.

It doesn't matter what you order if you don't know what to do with the data.

Here are some tests for assessing thyroid function. This list is by no means a complete list of tests for Hashimoto's. We will discuss more tests in upcoming chapters.

Medication and Testing

One really important thing to understand is the impact of your thyroid hormone medication on your blood test results. When you test and how you test matters.

In my experience, most doctors say you don't need to fast to test your thyroid. As with most things we always need to ask whether or not that is true.

T3 has a relatively short half life, which means it is only active in the body for a few hours. T4, both synthetic and natural, has a much longer period of activity.

A study by Scobbo et al in 2004 called *Serum TSH variability in normal individuals: the influence of time of sample collection* showed that TSH results declined in 97 of the 100 people studied by an average of 23.39% when compared to early morning, fasting TSH results. So testing later in the day may result in lower TSH than early in the morning.

Bottom line? Test your levels first thing in the morning, before taking medication and fast before doing so. This will give you the most accurate reading.

Top 7 Thyroid Tests

Here is a good summary of some of the most important thyroid tests to take to your doctor if you suspect that you have Hashimoto's.

If you already know you have Hashimoto's, retesting antibodies may not be a good measure of success or failure.

This is because antibody levels are always changing and the number of the test result really represents a "snap shot" of that moment in time only.

They can be helpful to spot larger trends and to see if a given treatment strategy is having an effect on antibody numbers, but they should not be the primary focus of testing, in my opinion.

For an in depth discussion on antibodies and antibody testing please visit the supplemental area of our website: https://hashimotos-diet.com/roadmap-to-remission-supplemental/

Make sure you request a copy of your thyroid labs so that you can see them yourself and so that you can double check to make sure they were interpreted correctly.

- TSH (Thyroid Stimulating Hormone)
- Free T3
- Free T4
- Reverse T3
- Thyroid peroxidase antibodies (TPO antibodies)
- Thyroglobulin antibodies (TG antibodies)
- Thyroid ultrasound

2. P = Prioritize and Plan

From the data, determine where the issues are and what areas need improvement. Are you converting properly? Is there enough thyroid hormone in the body? Is it being absorbed?

Compare symptoms to lab test results. If they are inconsistent, something may not be working. Create a plan based on the data. If you don't know how to do this, this is precisely the place to get help.

It is highly recommended that you keep things simple to keep variables to a minimum and that you keep a daily food and activity journal to identify patterns and successful results.

3. A =Act & Adapt:

There are many potential courses of action. Let's look at some foods, vitamins and minerals that improve thyroid hormone conversion.

Important minerals and supplements for proper thyroid function include:

- **Zinc**—Needed to form TSH and too little can impair T4 to T3 conversion.

- **Selenium**—Acts as a catalyst to convert T4 to T3 and helps protect that body from oxidative damage.

- **Magnesium**—Proper thyroid function depends on a fine balance between calcium and magnesium. Magnesium is also used by the body in more than three hundred enzyme reactions.

- **Iron**—Adequate amounts of iron are necessary to transport T3 to the cells of your body. Being even "a little anemic" is not acceptable.

- **Iodine**—A controversial nutrient, to say the least. Important for proper thyroid function, but excessive iodine can cause significant problems with people with Hashimoto's.

- **Glutathione:** One of the most beneficial antioxidants in the body. See below for a more detailed explanation of all the good things it does.

Food Sources for Needed Vitamins and Minerals

The following list of vitamins, minerals and supplements may, of course, also be taken in supplement form. I've gathered food sources of all of them because I'd like you to get in the habit of seeing your diet as your first choice for treatment and healing.

Here are some food sources with these nutrients. Note: some of the foods on this list like the nuts, seeds and grains may not be appropriate for some people with Hashimoto's. We will discuss more on diet in the chapter on the Earth Element.

- **Zinc**—oysters, herring, liver, oatmeal, maple syrup, brewer's yeast, sunflower seeds, soybeans, mushrooms, sardines, pecans, pumpkin seeds

- **Selenium**—brazil nuts, brown rice, brewer's yeast, eggs, garlic, liver

- **Magnesium**—kelp, almonds, cashews, brazil nut, dulse, peanut, walnut, filbert, sesame seed, lima beans, peas, millet

- **Iron**—dulse, kelp, rice bran, pumpkin seeds, beans, lentil, parsley, walnut, apricot, almond, raisins, swiss chard, spinach, dates, fig, kale, cucumber, cauliflower, cabbage

- **Iodine**—kelp, dulse, agar, swiss chard, turnip greens, summer squash, mustard greens, watermelon, cucumber, spinach, asparagus, kale, turnip

- **Glutathione**—Consume sulfur-rich foods. The main ones in the diet are garlic, onions, and the cruciferous vegetables (broccoli, kale, collards, cabbage, cauliflower, watercress, etc). Take glutathione or N-Acetyl-Cysteine.

Hypothyroidism Nutrition

- Beware of the "ides" Avoid fluoride, bromide and chloride and Chlorine (fluoride can be found in many toothpastes, bromide in fire retardants and furniture and fluoride and chlorine in tap water), since these elements may block the iodine receptors in the thyroid glands, leading to reduced hormone production and eventually hypothyroidism. Drink steam-distilled water or reverse Osmosis water only.

- Avoid gluten, dairy, and soy 100 percent. All three have been found to aggravate autoimmunity, increase thyroid tissue destruction, and decrease availability of thyroid hormone in the body.

- Encourage the consumption of foods (or supplements) rich in vitamin B complex to promote the proper generation and utilization of energy.

Here are some food sources of B Vitamins:

- **Vitamin B1**—rice bran, sunflower seeds, pinto beans, peas, lentils, almonds, turnip greens, collard greens, kale, asparagus

- **Vitamin B2**—salmon, trout, cod, mackerel, perch, oysters, mushrooms, almonds, hijiki

- **Vitamin B3**—rice bran, red pepper, wild rice, kelp, sesame seed, peaches, brown rice, mushrooms, barley, almonds, apricot

- **Vitamin B5 (Pantothenic Acid)**—beef, chicken, salmon, mackerel, sardines, barley, rice, avocado, plums, raisins, almonds, dates

- **Vitamin B6**—banana, barley, brewer's yeast, molasses, brown rice, liver, beef, cabbage, carrots, potato, yams

- **Vitamin B12:** beef liver, beef kidney, ham, sole, scallops, eggs, oats, pickles, amasake, algae, spirulina and chlorella, brewer's yeast

- **Folic Acid:** liver, asparagus, lima beans, spinach, swiss chard, kale, cabbage, sweet corn

Don't Believe the Hype

The Research on Goitrogens

People with Hashimoto's and those with low thyroid function (which is commonly seen with other autoimmune diseases) are often told to avoid cruciferous vegetables, spinach, radishes, peaches, and strawberries because of their goitrogenic properties.

"Goitrogen" is a word that was coined in the 1950s to describe something that causes the formation of a goiter, also knows as an enlarged thyroid gland.

The term has multiple meanings and can be anything from thyroid hormone suppression, to changing the way thyroid hormone is produced in the body to slowing the rate of absorption of iodine.

With cruciferous vegetables, they have been called "goitrogenic" because they have the potential to block iodine absorption.

This was a problem in the 1950s, when iodine deficiency was a much more common cause of hypothyroidism. Back then, lower iodine levels were much more of problem from a public health stand point.

Well, this is 2015, and the world has changed. Today, our world is awash with environmental toxins, radiation, and plastics, all of which are much more important health threats, in my opinion.

The Research Doesn't Support This

Avoiding these foods is not well justified and is not supported by research. According to Sarah Ballantyne, PhD, scientist and researcher, in her book, The Paleo Approach, this family of vegetables is a great source of a group of sulfur-containing compounds called glucosinolates.

When these vegetables are chewed or chopped, the enzyme myrosinase in these plants breaks the glucosinolates apart into different compounds, many of which are potent antioxidants that prevent cancer. Two of them—isothiocyanates and thiocyanates—are also known goitrogens.

Isothiocyanates and thiocyanates seem to reduce thyroid function by inhibiting the action of the enzyme thyroid peroxidase (also known as thyroid peroxidase or TPO).

As described in the previous chapter, during thyroid hormone synthesis, TPO is the enzyme that uses iodine to produce either T4 thyroid protein hormone (Thyroxine) or the more active T3 thyroid hormone.

When isothiocyanates or thiocyanates are consumed in large enough quantities, they can interfere with the function of the thyroid gland.

However, there is no evidence of a link between normal human consumption of these componds and thyroid pathogens unless you have iodine deficiency.

So, if you are severely deficient in iodine or selenium, addressing that deficiency before eating tons of cruciferous vegetables is a good idea. In fact, addressing these deficiencies is a good idea period.

The enzyme myrosinase is also deactivated by cooking, so cooked cruciferous vegetables can still be enjoyed while you're working on correcting any deficiencies. Steaming and blanching are both good ways to cook and preserve important compounds and phytonutrients.

Another important point to consider is that these vegetables have potent anti-cancer effects. Researchers Lee JH et al did a meta-analysis published in the European Journal of Endocrinology in December 2014. The link between Hashimoto's and papillary thyroid cancer was established but it is not fully understood if the inflammation from Hashimoto's causes the cancer or if the inflammation is the result of the cancer.

Furthermore, in the case of papillary thyroid cancer the presence of Hashimoto's means a better prognosis and lower risk of reoccurrence if you do develop thyroid cancer.

In any case, eliminating the benefit of these vegetables from our diets makes no sense because of their known anti-cancer effects. Also, in a recent clinical trial evaluating the safety of isothiocyanates isolated from broccoli sprouts, no adverse effects were reported (including no reductions in thyroid function).

And finally, small amounts of these thiocyanate compounds, like what you would get from including cruciferous vegetables in your diet, stimulate T4 synthesis, meaning that these vegetables labeled goitrogens actually support thyroid function.

Have These Foods with Selenium

A strong connection exists between isothiocyanates and selenium in the formation of other important enzymes for the thyroid (thioredoxin reductase and glutathione peroxidase).

Consuming isothiocyanates with selenium gives the body antioxidants that can provide a major boost to your defenses and help prevent cancer. So I advise you to eat more rather than less of these fruits and vegetables, even if you have Hashimoto's, as long as you're not deficient in iodine and selenium.

As with anything, moderation is always recommended. Don't eat wheel barrows full of cruciferous vegetables and don't live in fear of them.

Additional Considerations

TCM Food Perspective:

- According to TCM (Traditional Chinese Medicine), vegetables are generally cold in nature and meats are usually warm in property. Since individuals with hypothyroidism often have yang deficiency and cold presentations, increased consumption of meats (especially lamb) may help warm up the body and dispel cold.

Hyperthyroidism Nutrition:

- Avoid gluten, dairy, and soy 100 percent. All three have been found to aggravate autoimmunity, increase thyroid tissue destruction, and decrease availability of thyroid hormone in the body.

- Check your dosage of thyroid replacement hormone. One cause of hyperthyroid symptoms may be too much medication. Another maybe related to the adrenals, we will explore that when we get to the Water Element. Sometimes people have mixed presentations where they have both hypo and hyper symptoms. This can be the result of too much thyroid hormone in the system that isn't getting absorbed equally throughout the body.

- Consider doing more to address autoimmunity. Cutting out gluten, dairy, and soy are important first steps, but may not be enough. You may need to address autoimmunity more aggressively by adopting an elimination diet or the **Autoimmune Paleo Approach.** We will explore this further in the Chapters on the Earth Element.

Qi Gong Exercise for the Thyroid

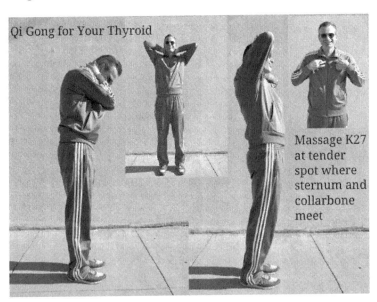

Qi Gong for Your Thyroid

Massage K27 at tender spot where sternum and collarbone meet

Here is a simple exercise that is very beneficial for the thyroid.

Neck Squeeze: You may do this exercise sitting or standing. Relax, close your eyes and interlace your hands behind your neck. Then let your head hang forward and allow the weight of your arms to gently stetch your neck muscles. After that, bring your elbows close together in front of your face, squeezing the sides of your neck with the heels of your hands.

Inhale slowly and deeply, raising your head as you gently bring your bent elbows out to the sides, life your head up and let it gently tilt back. Exhale slowly and repeat the whole movement again.

Repeat this breathing exercise for two to five minutes; then continue with the next exercise that involves the use of the acupuncture point K 27.

K 27 Meditation: This acupuncture point is located in the tender triangle where your sternum and collarbone meet.

Close your eyes, take slow deep breaths as you slowly let your head turn from side to side. Visualize your entire neck region relaxing as you continue to breathe deeply, and gently applying pressure or tapping on these points.

Gently let your head tilt backwards, forwards and slowly rotate while visualizing blood flowing peacefully into through your thyroid and the area that surrounds it. Completely let go and relax.

Then sit quietly and meditate for 5 minutes, visualizing your thyroid healing and regenerating.

4. R = Reassess & Readjust

Execute your plan and then reevaluate in one to two weeks. If you don't feel any better, then reassess. If you feel some improvement, try to determine what led to it and do more of that.

In order to do this properly, you need to establish a baseline to begin with. Keep a journal, note where you began, then re-evaluate and compare.

Clinical Pearl:

One important area to reassess is your reaction to thyroid replacement hormone if you are taking it. Not everyone has the same reaction, for a variety of reasons.

And also, there's no such thing as a "bad" reaction. Everything is a test and every outcome, whether it's what we wanted or not, provides valuable information.

Here's a quick breakdown of what reactions to different types of thyroid hormone therapy may mean:

Felt Better With Bio-Identicals (Like Armour, Westhroid, etc.)

Some people truly do feel better with bio-identicals. It's not true of everyone but the addition of T3 can sometimes be the answer because these people:

May need T3 due to problems with the thyroid hormone receptors on cells

Were unable to convert T4 to T3 when using T4-only medication

Had sensitivities to dyes or fillers in synthetic compounds that are not in bio-identical compounds

Have receptor sites on cells that simply respond better to bio-identical than synthetic hormones

Did Better With T3 Only

Some people improve with the addition of T3, while others do their best with T3 only. And these can be synthetic or bio-identical.

This can happen for a couple of reasons:

Their receptor sites are resistant to thyroid hormone because of high cortisol, high homocysteine, inflammation, low progesterone, vitamin A deficiency and more.

They have difficulty converting T4 to T3

Didn't Feel Better With T3 or Bio-identical Hormones

In both cases, more T3 is introduced.

These people may not have too little T3, they have an active and uncontrolled autoimmune process causing the release of thyroid hormone.

These are also the people who often vacillate from hyper to hypo. They have an immune flare up, more hormone is released and then they crash, it calms done and they are hypo again.

In some cases, these people can have excess adrenal hormones (i.e., epinephrine) caused by too much nicotine, caffeine, stress or exercising too much.

Feel Better on Synthetic Hormones

Some people actually feel better on synthetic hormones.

These can be people who are converting well, have an overactive metabolism and just don't need more T3.

These are people who also really benefit from an approach that will calm the autoimmune attacks that cause their thyroid to be revved up in the first place.

Feel Fatigued and Run Down

This reaction is sometimes discounted, but it can also be meaningful.

These people may be sensitive to the ingredients and fillers.

If they are taking bi-oidentical hormones and they have this reaction, they may have an autoimmune response to the replacement hormone.

To learn more about thyroid replacement hormone visit the supplemental area on our website: www.hashimotos-diet.com/r2rsupplemntal

5. T = Try & Try Again

Double down on what worked. Change what didn't. Don't give up if at first you didn't get earth shattering results.

This is an ongoing process; your goal should be on building long term success.

Also, be sure to keep track of what you did and worked, take time to celebrate it and understand it and then build on those successes.

It's remarkable how often people try things without first establishing, in an organized and systematic way, where they are.

Climbing a mountain doesn't happen all at once, you get to the top one step at a time. Every step forward is a small victory that you can build on.

Make sure you stay conscious of them as best you can.

It is often these little victories that lead to more profound changes because they lead to a change of momentum.

Chapter Six

The Metal Element:
Balancing the Immune System

In this chapter we're going to cover something that is fascinating but poorly understood—the immune system—which is the Metal element in Chinese medicine.

You'll learn how Hashimoto's affects the immune system as well as some powerful steps for restoring balance.

You'll also discover some common triggers that can cause flare ups and immune dysfunction.

Finally, we'll look at testing the immune system and what to do with that data.

Okay, let's start with the big picture.

What Does the Immune System Do?

The immune system protects the body from foreign invaders. Its like the body's military. It finds the bad guys (like bacteria, fungus, parasites, and viruses) and it kills them. It also cleans things up by destroying dead and dying cells.

This is called cellular apoptosis, and if this process stops working, cancer develops. In addition, the immune system creates inflammation as part of the process of healing after an injury.

It is amazingly plastic and adaptive, meaning it's always changing. It continually confounds researchers because it doesn't follow simplistic logic. It can't afford to; it must constantly defend us from so many types of invaders, literally trillions of foreign invaders in a lifetime.

Recent research in fields such as Psychneuroimmunology has shown that immune system has the ability to communicate with the nervous system, the endocrine system, and digestive system, and that it is actively modulating and influencing the body all the time.

And it is not linear. Meaning, different parts of the immune system seem to do things in opposite directions at the same time. We'll look at some examples in a second.

And this can get more complicated and confusing when we're trying to understand autoimmune disease. Because people are also at different stages of progression, they have problems with various other systems, and they have different genetic profiles. It's no wonder that practitioners of all kinds are sometimes lost when it comes to dealing with autoimmunity.

The ancient Chinese described immunity and defense in the body as Wei qi. This defensive qi was thought of as brave and fierce, which it truly is.

And where is it in the body? Much of it found in the lymphatic system.

This is where the immune cells live and differentiate. They are born in the bone marrow and travel here to mature and do various different jobs.

And we have four primary barriers: the skin, the walls of the digestive tract, the lungs, and the blood-brain barrier. The lungs and the intestinal walls are heavily lined with lymph nodes because this is where a lot of invasions happen. They are airborne or they come with food.

The Immune System Has Many Parts

The immune system has many different parts, but the two important parts are called non-specific and specific immunity.

One theory of immune regulation involves homeostasis or balance between T-helper 1 (Th1) and T-helper 2 (Th2) activity. This is a very popular theory that has influenced many alternative care practitioners and treatment strategies.

As we have learned more about the immune system, the limitations of this theory have started to appear.

A Little Background on Th1 and Th2 Theory

TH-1 and TH-2 theory traces its origin back to research done on mice 1986. It was discovered that mouse T-helper cells expressed different kinds of immune proteins known as cytokines.

This theory was then applied to human immunity and it was determined that TH-1 and TH-2 cells directed responses through different pathways.

TH-1 cells were linked to fighting viruses, and other pathogens inside cells. They also helped kill cancer cells and cause certain types of skin reactions. You can think of them as yin.

TH-2 cells, on the other hand, affected antibody production and fought things outrside of cells. You can think of them as yang.

TH-2 Dominance

TH-2 dominance (which means a stronger relative presence than TH-1) is linked to the body's ability to tolerate transplanted tissue and the fetus during pregnancy. Normally the immune system attacks anything that is not 'self'.

A woman's body goes into TH-2 dominance temporarily during pregnancy. This is one of the possible explanations why some women have the onset of Hashimoto's after their pregnancy.

The temporary TH-2 dominance which balances the TH-1 attack on the thyroid recedes and the immune pendulum swings back to TH-1 and sometimes this happens with a vengeance. (Originally, the majority of people with Hashimoto's were thought to be TH-1 dominant, but this is an oversimplification and is not always the case.)

Over time we have come to learn that TH-1 and TH-2 are far more nueanced than orginally thought and their proteins sometimes behave in unexpected ways. So the theory has been shown to have inconsistencies and real life is not a textbook or a laboratory, so there are rarely TH-1 or TH-2 exclusive patterns.

We have also learned that other immune cells, like antigen-presentiing cells can also affect the immune system in similar ways to TH-1 and TH-2 cells. For example, another cytokine called IL-6 (Interleukin 6) is produced by dendritic cells in the intestines and it has been shown to promote TH-2 and to dampen TH-1.

Why does this matter? Elevated IL-6 has been linked to lower levels of T4 and T3 in the blood. Il-6 is commonly found the fat around the abdomen.

These different parts of the immune system can be rather confusing. The important thing to understand is that a delicate balance between the yin and yang aspects of the immune system is our ultimate goal. You can't just attack this with a heavy hand and try to shut down one side or the other or over-stimulate either side.

Instead we must work to bring balance and harmony because many of the diseases (like Hashimoto's) that were considered to be exclusively TH-1 or TH-2 domnant have been shown not to be when examined more closely.

Furthermore, in some experiments, TH-1 dominance has actually been shown to become transformed into TH-2 dominance throught the depletion of glutathione. So it's not always a good idea to simply push one side or the other. You might wind up with unintended consequences.

Much like real life, this theory isn't perfect. But it is a helpful framework for understanding the amazingly complex world that is our immune system. Let's take a look at some of these TH-1 and TH-2 proteins more closely.

Non-Specific Immunity

The non-specific immune system is our immediate attack response. These are the front line soldiers that hang out in our borders (the mucous membranes of our lungs, digestive tract, skin, and brain) and kill invaders.

This part of our immune system is called the T-Helper 1 (or Th1) response. These are the macrophages (the Pac-man cells) and Killer T cells (the elite squads) that are pathogen-killing machines.

Th1 is also broken down into messenger proteins like Interleukin-12 (IL 12), Interleukin 2 (IL-2), Interferon Gamma (IFN) and Tumor Necrosis Factor (TNF). **These are the bad-ass Navy Seals that get the job done.**

IL-12 is a commander and facilitator that provokes inflammation. It's responsible for helping natural killer cells mature and is also involved in turning on genes that result in attacks on specific organs and it stimulates the TH-1 response. It has been implicated as an important player in Hashimoto's attacks on the thyroid.

IL-2 is synthesized by CD 4 T cells, which then enables increased antibody production and improved bone marrow responses to other immune cells.

A close relative of IL-2, IL-15, has been shown to be low in Hashimoto's, and treatment with levothyroxine can increase IL-15 levels, as do some Chinese herbs (see the last chapter in the Metal Element).

Again, here is the contradictory nature of the immune system. Increasing IL-15, some theorize, may reduce the destruction of thyroid cells in Hashimoto's. Yet many people thought that with Hashimoto's, Th1 was too strong. You see? Yang within yin. Yin and yang theory can help us understand contradictions in the immune system.

Tumor Necrosis Factor (TNF), TNF alpha, kills tumor cells. It turns on angiogenesis (the hallmark of malignant tumors), promotes fibroblasts, and is involved in wound healing.

Drugs called biologic response modifiers, or "biologics," block the action of TNF alpha. These have grown in popularity in recent years and are used by some rheumatologists to treat autoimmune diseases.

The downside of this type of therapy is that it makes you very vulnerable to certain kinds of life threatening infections, like tuberculosis.

TNF beta is another commander who helps kill tumor cells, activates genes, and mediates CD8 T cells, NK cells, and helper-killer T cells to induce them to fatally injure their targets.

A TNF receptor called CD95, which is responsible for cell death, has been found to be very high in patients with Hashimoto's. It's a factor in the destruction of thyroid tissue.

Specific Immunity

The specific immune system produces antibodies that label the bad guys. This part of the immune system is like the C.I.A. It gathers intelligence on the bad guys and it labels them with an antibody.

Once an antibody labels a foreign invader, it's much easier for the killer cells to destroy it. And like the C.I.A., it takes a while for them to gather the intelligence, so this process is usually delayed for a period of time.

This part of the immune system is called T-Helper 2 (or Th2). These cells also do more than just label, they also attach themselves to certain cells like viruses to keep them from entering into our cells. This is important because once they are in our cells, they are much harder to kill, and they can replicate more quickly.

Th2 is also broken down into interleukins. IL-10 and IL-4 are two important ones.

IL-10 has been implicated in numerous autoimmune disease, such as type I diabetes and multiple sclerosis. But it is a perfect example of the unpredictability of the immune system. It turns on some immune functions and shuts off others. It can block IL-1, IL-6, and TNF alpha, but turns on IL-2 and IL-4.

And to further complicate matters, research has now shown that IL-10 is produced by and down regulates the function of both TH-1 and TH-2.

IL-4 is produced by CD 4 T cells and activates IgE, an immunoglobin important for creating immunity to parasites and involved in allergies.

Complicated, But Really Cool

To further complicate matters we have other parts of the immune system driving the immune attack, and this is the family of interleukins that belong to IL-1. IL-1 is released by the pac-man cells that are the frontline attackers.

IL-18 belongs in this family of cells and a lot of it is in Hashimoto's patients, especially those with severe symptoms that don't respond to levothyroxine treatment. It may be responsible for severe inflammation.

Both parts of the immune system are needed for certain types of invaders. For example, viruses are often very small and can sneak past the border security.

Next, the Th2 system uses its cellular informants to sniff the viruses out and it tags them. This can take several days to initiate and is why it takes most people a few days to recover from the common cold, which is caused by a virus.

In a general sense, the Th1 system is considered inflammatory, and the Th2 system is considered anti-inflammatory. But in reality, they are both involved in the process of inflammation.

And IL-12 and IL-18 are important drivers of inflammation in Hashimoto's.

New Research Has Revealed Other Parts of the Immune System

Recent research has shown that there are other parts of the immune system that also play important roles in this process. T-Helper 3 (Th3) or T reg (T regulatory) cells are a part of the immune system that can calm and dampen other more aggressive cells and proteins.

T3 cells are kind of like the generals of the immune system. They call back the troops once they've attacked and keep them disciplined so they don't pillage and attack the entire body.

TH-3 cells are like the generals of the immune system

This part of the immune system plays an important role in autoimmune disease and must be strengthened and balanced. Both Vitamin D and glutathione have been found to be quite helpful in doing this.

In addition, TH-3 cells may actually have a different origin than Th1 and Th2. They seem to come from dendritic cells in the intestines.

Another type of immune cell is T-Helper 17 (Th17). These cells are instigators and they rev up the attack and can make the damage and the carnage much more intense. A delicate balance of all parts of the immune system is important and with an autoimmune disease like Hashimoto's, this balance is lost.

What Happens with Hashimoto's?

In most cases of Hashimoto's some combination of factors (virus, environmental toxins, genetics, gluten, breakdown of the intestinal lining and so forth) lead to a slow, gradual attack against the thyroid.

This reaction eventually leads to the loss of enough thyroid cells that the condition presents as hypothyroidism and is seen on a blood test as high TSH.

TSH becomes high because, as we have learned, when the thyroid is not working properly, the pituitary gland increases production of TSH to increase thyroid gland activity. For some people with Hashimoto's, the thyroid doesn't develop overactive symptoms. Over time, they develop symptoms of low thyroid function and are put on thyroid replacement hormone.

For others, periods of hyperactivity can occur. They may vacillate between hyper and hypo symptoms. These people may develop behavioral issues that resemble bipolar disorder.

In some cases, however, patients can develop full blown hyperthyroidism and Graves' disease (also a thyroid autoimmune disease). There are even some patients who have a confirmed diagnosis of both Hashimoto's and Graves' disease.

Autoimmunity Is Ignored While TSH Is Managed

For many people, the issue of the autoimmune attack is never addressed. Instead, these patients are considered to be properly managed by having normalized TSH. In reality, these people are having their TSH managed, but the underlying problem is not being addressed.

Over time, they lose more and more thyroid cells and they need more thyroid replacement hormone. The result, for many people, is that they continue to have all the hypothyroid symptoms (like fatigue, hair loss, depression, constipation, and cold hands and feet) because the root cause has been largely ignored.

Since the thyroid is being destroyed, there is less thyroid hormone production. The immune system needs thyroid hormones to modulate Th1 and Th2 activity, so when this happens, the immune system can short circuit. This leads to a larger number of T cells, and auto-antibody producing B cells. These cells accumulate in the thyroid and kill thyroid cells.

There are many possible scenarios that can lead to this outcome. Dr. Datis Kharrazian, D.C. in his book, *Why Do I Still Have Thyroid Symptoms?*, gives us some excellent examples of scenarios that can lead to this.

* The T suppressor (Th3) cells that regulate the immune response could be too few in number, and like a weak general that has lost control of his troops, this can lead to unchecked attacks by the immune system. And tissue like the thyroid becomes a casualty.

*Th1 has a number of different soldiers, these are the interleukins we just discussed. These all have specific jobs. For example, interleukin 2 (IL-2) is a messenger chemical that sends out orders for the killer cells to start killing.

Some people make too much IL-2 and this creates a frenzy of destruction that can lead to the death of the thyroid cells. Chronic viral infections can cause too much IL-2 to be made and have been linked to the development of autoimmune thyroid disease. In fact, in the patient population that I have worked with about 75% of the people I have seen have some history of exposure to the Epstein Barr virus. IL-2 may be a reason why.

* TH2 also has lots of different soldiers. Interleukin 4 (IL-4) deploys B cells. Like some rouge C.I.A. agents, these cells can go crazy and tag the wrong proteins, and destruction of thyroid tissue is the result. Parasites and food allergies can cause too much IL-4 to be made.

* Too much sugar can cause the body to rapidly release insulin. These spikes in insulin can stimulate the production of too many B cells, they start tagging too many things, and this can lead to destruction of the thyroid.

Sugar imbalances can have a big impact on immune function.

And this is just the tip of the iceberg. In reality, there are many variables and many potential reasons for the immune system to short circuit. This is what makes treatment and management so challenging. And this is also why you must have a multi-pronged approach.

Initially, researchers thought Hashimoto's was a Th-1 dominant disease (but this is not true for everyone and has proven to be an oversimplification).

It seems IL-18 and IL-12 also act together to cause more destruction to the thyroid. Look for development of drugs that inhibit these two interleukins.

Hashimoto's people also often have a weak Th3 regulatory system and their Th2 may or may not be out of control. Th17 is also often wound up, making the attack more intense.

And none of this happens in a vacuum. This is all taking place in the context of the body where the immune system is interacting with the endocrine system, the digestive system, and the nervous system.

Talk about complicating the task of unwinding this mess; it's no wonder patients and doctors alike get frustrated and overwhelmed.

OK, whew! That's a lot of interleukins!

Recap of Immune System and Hashimoto's

1. Th1/Th2 balance is a theory that was really popular and is now less popular because these relationships are a bit more nuanced than originally thought. But it is still useful and can help treatment if you can identify imbalances.

These two parts of the immune system have a kind of yin and yang relationship, so strengthening one can sometimes help calm the other.

Th1 is like the Navy Seals. They are the frontline attackers.

Th2 is like the CIA. They gather intelligence on the bad guys.

2. IL-18 and IL-12 are bad guys, and we want to calm them down.

3. Th17 is a troublemaker that does both good and bad stuff. But, generally, we want to calm it down too.

4. Th3 is the command and control center, kind of like a general. This is often weak in Hashimoto's folks. Making the general stronger can really be beneficial therapeutically.

We'll discuss how to influence all these different parts of the immune system shortly.

How the Immune System and Thyroid Are Connected in Hashimoto's

Before we go further, let's review a little from the last chapter and see how it relates to this chapter.

As you recall, we looked at the thyroid, so let's highlight a few of the important takeaways.

1. There may be "functional hypothyroidism" or sufficient thyroid hormone that isn't getting into the cells of the body.

This is a situation in which you can have normal TSH (in the pituitary) and normal T4 and still feel like crap.

I put this question to our Facebook support group and got over 350 comments (at last count). The overwhelming majority of people said that they had normal TSH, T4 and a host of hypothyroid symptoms (fatigue, brain fog and memory issues, weight issues, constipation, anxiety and depression, hair loss, brittle hair and nails, etc.)

Why? Many reasons, but one is that TSH is made in the pituitary, and the pituitary absorbs and responds to thyroid hormone differently than other cells in the body.

Add to this all the accompanying problems that are involved in Hashimoto's, like systemic inflammation, digestive problems, a poorly functioning liver, and the stress of life on top of having to deal with this and what do you get?

2. The perfect recipe for diminished sensitivity and absorption of thyroid hormone into your cells.

The best way to find out is to test T3 or free T3 and rT3, then to divide T3 by rT3. If the ratio is too low (low T3 and high rT3), then you may have a state of hypothyroidism in your cells. T4 can be elevated in these cases also.

This is also sometimes called **low T3 syndrome**. Taking T3 may or may not help. As with everything involving Hashimoto's, there is no magic bullet. You have to evaluate everything first and then try some things.

Inflammation, chronic stress, and autoimmune disease attacking other things (like the pituitary and other parts of the brain) can all cause low T3 syndrome and functional hypothyroidism.

And this state of too little T3 can have a big impact on the immune system.

Thyroid hormones play a very important role in the growth, formation and balance of immune cells. Every single immune cell has receptor sites for thyroid hormones. Immune cells need thyroid hormone to mature and to regulate TH-1 and TH-2 proteins and cells.

It's all connected, people.

Yao et al found that shown that T4 may calm inflammatory proteins like IL-10 and IL-4 in mice. And other researchers have found evidence of the same to be true on human subjects. As we saw above, when these cells get out of control this can mean more inflammation, more pain and destruction of thyroid tissue.

Essentially, thyroid hormone is like the voice of reason for the angry mob of immune cells and proteins. It gets everyone to just chill out and relax.

So we clearly have the makings of a vicious cycle here. Right? One problem reinforcing another.

Immune system imbalance can lead to more inflammation which can prevent thyroid hormone from being absorbed properly and this leads to functional hypothyroidism and thyroid receptor issues and back and forth they go. They create a positive feedback loop, reinforcing each other and making each other worse. And the result is definitely not positive.

To make matters worse, thyroid hormone also has a major impact on inflammation in the intestines. It is one of the things that keeps the cell walls in the intestines strong. It also stimulates gastric cells and intestinal walls cells and hypothyroidism can lead to leaky gut or intestinal permeability. This is a breakdown of the walls of the intestines. (We will explore this in detail in an upcoming chapter.)

So, you see, we have a problem here. Two important factors are constantly creating circumstances in the body that are continuing to make Hashimoto's worse. These are two children with some serious issues!

Important Takeaway:

The most important takeaway here is that, while thyroid hormone can help autoimmune dysfunction, just throwing more thyroid hormone at the problem may not be the answer.

If you don't address the underlying autoimmunity, you'll just be spinning your wheels because the process of autoimmunity can create this state of functional hypothyroidism, which is a major factor in the downward spiral and progression of this disease.

Why is Autoimmunity So Often Ignored in Hashimoto's?

It's important to understand that Hashimoto's is much more than just a thyroid disorder. It is an autoimmune disease that involves multiple systems of the body. Let's take a look now at how autoimmune disease is handled in today's healthcare system.

Well, first, we see a huge void in our healthcare model for treating, managing and, even, properly understanding this condition. Because so little is understood, we have basically no specialist for autoimmune disease.

Think about it. Who do you see? A rhuematologist? Maybe. And what do they do? They prescribe prednisone and other immunosuppressive agents (i.e., biologics like Enbrel).

Their goal? It is to completely suppress and weaken the immune system or block one aspect of the immune system from functioning properly. That's pretty much it.

In my own personal experience I'll never forget the moment I realized that there was not going to be anything done until things got "bad enough". Holy crap! We are on our own in the conventional medical model, especially in an early to moderate stage of tissue destruction.

Doing Nothing Is Not Acceptable

Often nothing is done until there is significant destruction in the body. If you're living with it, that's too late, in my opinion. This approach leads to a significant loss in quality of life, which for some means they can't work, and they can't spend time with their family and friends.

Why isn't more attention being given to autoimmunity? When you look at the sheer number of cases, it's virtually epidemic.

According to the American Autoimmune Related Disease Association, one out of every twelve men and one out of every nine women have autoimmune disease.

And the numbers are higher than other major diseases: the NIH (National Institute of Health) thinks that up to 23.5 million Americans have autoimmune disease. Just to compare, an estimated 9 million have cancer, and 22 million have heart disease.

This is especially crazy when you understand how autoimmune disease is defined. An autoimmune disease is officially recognized when about 70–90 percent of the target disease is destroyed. You don't just go from 0–70 percent destruction overnight.

Why aren't more people talking about this? Is it because it's not life threatening?

Autoimmune Disease Can Be Life Threatening

No. The stakes are really high here. Actually, autoimmune disease is one of the top ten leading causes of death in female children and women in all age groups up to sixty-four years of age.

I don't want to frighten you, but I want you to understand what the stakes are, so that you take this part of Hashimoto's seriously. And this comes into play when you have to decide what you are going to do.

In my personal and professional experience, the most effective changes are dietary and lifestyle changes and some of them are big, major changes for some people. When you see the big picture and the potential for where this can go and how destructive this can be, it makes not eating foods like gluten and dairy a no-brainer. That's not that big a sacrifice when your life is on the line.

I also want you to understand that these suggestions aren't some fad. They're being made because the risks of the status quo, of doing nothing or letting this disease progress unchecked, are just too high.

I'm really passionate about this for one simple reason. I've seen where this can progress and I hope this information can help some of you make changes in your life to prevent that.

Now, let's take a look at how Hashimoto's and autoimmunity can advance deeper into the body

Autoimmune disease can progresses in 2 different ways. Firstly, it goes deeper and deeper into the body causing more and more loss of function and the breakdown of other major systems. Secondly, it can progress onto other autoimmune diseases.

Three Stages of Autoimmune Disease

According to a number of researchers such as Arvin Parvathaneni, Daniel Fischman, Pramil Cheriyath, and Datis Kharrazian, DC, autoimmune disease is also a progressive disease that goes through three stages. While these are not recognized by the general medical community, they are very useful clinically.

As I stated above, autoimmune disease is not officially recognized until close to 70–90 percent of the target tissue is destroyed.

Well, wouldn't it be better to have some other way to identify these diseases before they destroy the target tissue? Before you've lost your ability to function and live and work like a normal person? For my way of thinking the answer is YES!

Stage 1: Silent Autoimmunity

In this stage, the body has lost tolerance to its own tissue, but there are no symptoms yet and it doesn't really affect the way that the system functions. This stage can, however, be identified by lab tests that show elevated antibodies. People can stay in this stage for years.

This is the best place to begin some sort of treatment aimed at prevention because your odds of getting good results are highest.

Physiologically, in this stage thyroid specific antigens are presented to antigen presenting cells (APCs) by thyroid cells, often after some kind of insult or environmental stressor(s). (For example, infection(s), excessive iodine, pregnancy, toxins in cigarette smoke, etc.)

95

Stage 2: Autoimmune Reactivity

In this stage, the destruction of the target tissue has begun. Elevated antibodies and some symptoms appear. However, the destruction is not significant enough to actually be labeled autoimmune disease because 70–90 percent of the target tissue has not yet been destroyed. This stage is where a lot of Hashimoto's patients are.

They may or may not have been placed on thyroid replacement hormone and that may or may not have normalized their thyroid lab results. However, the destructive autoimmune process is active and is progressing.

This is a very important stage for treating the immune dysfunction because you have a greater chance to slow or stop the destruction of that tissue and slow the progression to other autoimmune diseases.

Physiologically, this is the stage where APCs (Antigen Presnting Cells) differentiate into T cells and B cells and begin the process of destruction.

Stage 3: Autoimmune Disease

This stage is where Western medicine finally acknowledges the autoimmune disease. And it takes this long because you need significant destruction of tissue in order to see the destruction with an MRI or ultrasound.

Other findings include elevated antibodies, serious and significant symptoms, lab results, and special studies that all confirm a loss of function. Unfortunately, this is really late in the game. With Hashimoto's, this stage is where the thyroid is almost completely destroyed.

Luckily, most people don't reach this stage before they have been given thyroid replacement hormone because the symptoms have already become so serious that they will have sought out a doctor to help them before they got here.

Finally, this is the stage, physiologically, where positive feedback has led to massive destruction of the thyroid gland and major loss of function in other systems of the body. T cells have induced cytotoxicity, and B cells have produced antibodies that have led to apoptosis or programmed cell death of thyroid cells, and macrophages have infiltrated the thyroid and started producing the interleukin proteins we spoke about earlier.

The second type of progression is the progression to other autoimmune diseases.

Other Common Autoimmune Diseases Linked to Hashimoto's

According to a study from the UK published in the American Journal of Medicine in 2010, 14.3 percent of Hashimoto's patients had another autoimmune disease, with rheumatoid arthritis being the most common.

This was of a group of 495 patients with confirmed Hashimoto's. I also put the question to our Facebook group and we had over 122 responses from people who had Hashimoto's and one or more additional autoimmune disease.

In my opinion, every Hashimoto's patient and every doctor who treats them should be asking the question: "Where else is it?" In an upcoming chapter we'll look at some testing that can help you answer this question.

To read a more in depth discussion of other common autoimmune diseases that accompany Hashimoto's, visit the supplemental material section on our website.https://hashimotos-diet.com/roadmap-to-remission-supplemental/

What Causes Autoimmune Disease and Hashimoto's?

There is no single cause. In many people there is some exposure to a virus or other pathogen. For example, Epstein Barr virus (or other herpes viruses), Coxsackie virus, or other pathogen like Salmonella or Lyme disease. One theory is that these viral fragments may resemble thyroid tissue and that may be why the immune system attacks the thyroid after fighting the virus. This is known as molecular mimicry.

There may also be exposure to environmental toxins (mercury, bisphenol A, etc.), and these actually form what are called "neo-antigens." These new antigens comprise the chemical plus our own tissue.

The formation of these neo-antigens initiates an immune response, which may result in antibody production against the chemical and the human tissue hybrid. Continued exposure to the chemical and the production of antibodies against various tissue antigens may result in autoimmune reactivity.

A genetic component is also a factor with Hashimoto's. We often see clusters with family members. It is not unusual to find first degree relatives with thyroid disease with people who have confirmed Hashimoto's.

And we also know that exposure to gluten can be factor in the formation of autoimmune disease.

Gluten Sensitivity, Celiac Disease and Thyroid Autoimmunity Are Related

Celiac Disease and autoimmune thyroid disorders share a common genetic link, namely, the DQ2 allele.

This is a subtype of a region of cells called the HLA (or Human Leucocyte Antigen) System.

There is a region on cells located on some of our genes. Many of these are located on chromosome 6 (for those of you keeping count).

Mutations or defects of HLA have been linked to many different autoimmune diseases.

Exactly what happens is not known, there are numerous theories, but the end result is that our own tissue gets attacked and destroyed by the immune system.

With Celiac disease and autoimmune thyroid diseases we see an increase in both types of antibodies that lead to attack on these tissues.

Collin et al found 5.4% of 335 adult celiac patients, of whom 83% complied with a gluten-free diet, had autoimmune thyroid disease (autoimmune hypothyroidism or Graves' disease).

Counsell et al found that 14% of celiac patients had thyroid disorders. The same authors also noted a high prevalence of thyroglobulin antibodies (11%) and thyroid microsomal (TPO) antibodies (15%) in their CD patients.

Likewise, Velluzzi et al found the prevalence of thyroid peroxidase antibodies to be higher in CD (29.7%) than in healthy controls (9.6%).

"Yes, But I Was Tested For Gluten Antibodies and The Tests Were Negative"

This is another area of misinformation. Most doctors test for 2-4 gluten antibodies.

Current testing for Gluten-Reactivity and Celiac disease (CD) includes serum IgG and IgA against gliadin and tissue transglutaminase-2 (tTG2).

These antibodies are measured against minor components of a wheat protein called alpha-gliadin.

Here's the thing, wheat consists of multiple proteins and peptides including, alpha-gliadin, omega-gliadin, glutenin, gluteomorphin, prodynorphin, and agglutinins.

And the important thing to understand is that any of these antigens can cause an immune response.

So, even if you tested negative to celiac, you could still have gluten sensitivity or silent celiac disease because you may not have tested for the right thing.

Which Came First, The Gluten or the Autoimmunity?

This is a really interesting question that is controversial and no one really knows.

But, here's what we do know.

Autoimmunity doesn't just happen for no reason. It is the result of a perfect storm of factors.

As mentioned above, there's genetics, exposure to a virus or other pathogen, exposure to toxic chemicals and all these cause antibodies to be produced and somehow you get the breakdown of the intestines.

Ground zero is the intestinal mucosa.

One theory is that gluten, which is sticky and invasive (like a thief who can get into anywhere it wants), gets into the intestines, into the spaces between the intestines (the tight junctions) and eventually into the bloodstream. Then the immune system kicks in.

Antigen presenting cells like macrophages (those Pac man cells that munch the bad guys) start attacking and they stimulate the T helper cells.

These are either TH-1 or Th-2 or both (as we have learned) and these lead to pro-inflammatory immune cells and proteins, more antibodies, cross reactions – generally, all hell breaking loose.

And, finally as this plays out and is repeated over and over again every time you eat a piece of bread, a pastry, some cake, a doughnut, etc. you are unknowingly pushing your body further and further into autoimmunity.

Your immune system is so juiced it doesn't know which way is up and eventually, you lose self tolerance.

And loss of self tolerance means the immune system starts attacking your own tissue.

Another problem caused by gluten is that it makes thyroid hormone less effective.

Celiac Disease Has A Major Impact on Thyroid Hormone Absorption

An interesting study published by the American Thyroid Association found "…This study examined 68 patients with Hashimoto's thyroiditis alone and 35 patients with Hashimoto's thyroiditis and celiac disease.

The average dose of levothyroxine needed to treat patients with Hashimoto's thyroiditis alone was lower than the average dose required to treat patients with Hashimoto's and celiac disease.

When the patients with celiac disease went on a gluten-free diet while staying on the same dose of thyroxine, their TSH level decreased, indicating that their absorption of thyroxine had improved."

Going gluten free improved thyroid hormone absorption for these people. And this is not only true for people with celiac disease.

Next, I'd like to share with an interesting case study that someone posted on our Facebook group recently that shows the remarkable effect that gluten and a strict gluten-free diet can have.

"From December until this past Thursday, I have brought my TPO down from >1300 (topping out the scales) to 8 (literally, 8). My doctor is dumbfounded. I have strictly eliminated gluten (with his acknowledgement) and that is IT.

However, when I say strict, I mean STRICT. He said there would be no way my numbers could change like that by elimination (he is a much older school doctor) and he wouldn't believe it until he sees it on paper. Well, he just saw it on paper and was almost speechless.

Also, my last ultrasound, this past Wednesday, showed no enlargement of my thyroid and barely any misshape. My numbers have plummeted since February to the farthest end of hyper that the scales will show..."

Lori K 4/4/15

Commentary: This is a story and an outcome that is quite commonplace. For some, gluten is a very serious player in the inflammation and attack on thyroid tissue. And for this patient, the change was so dramatic and the impact so great that she became hyperthyroid and had to discontinue her medication.

This is also something we see repeatedly in clinical practice. Gluten and dairy (lactose) can both block thyroid hormone absorption and in many cases, going gluten free will improve (sometimes dramatically) the performance of thyroid replacement hormone.

In fact, sometimes it is so effective that people must lower their dosage or risk going into a hyperthyroid state.

Stress Also Plays a Major Role

Stress can also play a major role in the expression and proliferation of autoimmune disease and Hashimoto's. And some large, stressful life event is often the last straw.

In a retrospective study from the Journal Autoimmune Review, 2008, they noted that "...many retrospective studies found that a high proportion (up to 80 percent) of patients reported uncommon emotional stress before disease onset. Unfortunately, not only does stress cause disease, but the disease itself also causes significant stress in the patients, creating a vicious cycle."

This is a hugely important point that we're going to explore in an upcoming chapter. Stress and autoimmune disease go together like gamblers and con men. They just seem to bring out the worst in each other.

Stressful life events can sometimes be the final straw in series of events and factors that lead to autoimmune disease.

Recap Of Factors Leading to Hashimoto's:

1. Exposure to a pathogen: Epstein barr, Yersenia, Coxsackie virus, Herpes virus, Lyme disease or other pathogens have been linked to the initiaon of thyroid autoimmunity.

2. Genetic susceptibility. Often there is a family history of thyroid disease.

3. Exposure to enviromental toxins like mercury or BPA (bisphenol A). The body forms "neo-antigens" or hybrids of our tissue and the toxic substance and the immune system attacks them.

4. Leaky gut or Intestinal permeability. The gut is ground zero for autoimmunity, if this breaks down and your barrier systems become compromised this can lead to the loss of self-tolerance.

5. Exposure to gluten. Gluten, itself can lead to thyroid autoimmunity.

6. Stress. A major stressful event or prolonged stress can lead to thyroid (and other types of) autoimmunity.

It's not just one thing. It's a collection of many things and it's not your fault. You just got dealt a bad hand. What matters now is how you play that hand.

NEXT, Let's take a look at the immune system from the Chinese medical perspective. But before we do, here's another Hashimoment.

HASHIMOMENT:
GRIEVING THE LOSS OF YOUR OLD LIFE

A really common theme among people who suffer from the debilitating effects of Hashimoto's is the struggle to accept what is the new normal.

According to Chinese medicine, one of the signs of a blocked thyroid was unwillingness to change.

Isn't that ironic? Hashimoto's forces us to change so much, sometimes!

Diet, habits, lifestyle, situations that no longer serve us.

When it starts to affect our lives, the temptation is to look at all the things we can't do anymore. And we may need to grieve the loss of that old life for a period of time.

Another irony is that in Chinese medicine, the negative emotion of the Metal Element is excessive grief or an inability to let go of the grief.

One way to get over this is to see that there is another way to look at it.

Like spring, you have an opportunity for a new life: one where you eat a healthy diet, do the things that serve you and let go of the stressful situations that were not good for you anyway.

Change, though difficult, can be a good thing.

Chapter Seven

The Chinese Medicine View
of the Metal Element

Now, let's get into the Chinese medical perspective. As I said at the beginning, one important organ system that is involved with the immune response is the Metal Element.

Remember when I was talking about this not being linear? Well, Chinese medicine is brilliantly constructed to account for this lack of step-by-step linearity.

By observing nature and creating theories about interactions in the body, the ancient Chinese were able to describe function in the body in the way that it actually happens.

They did this by layering these different theories in different directions and on many levels simultaneously. You can put several of these theories on top of each other.

Right? We've already looked at yin and yang. These ideas are repeated all over the earth and the universe: the moon, the sun, night, day, cold, hot, summer, winter, etc., *ad infinitum*. Yin, yang, yin, yang.

Then we have the 5 Elements: each of these have a yin and yang representative. In the Metal Element it's the lung that is yin and the large intestines that are yang. I was always puzzled by why. Why are these two systems connected? Well look at the lymphatic system. That's the connection. The immune system is what unites them.

Without getting too crazy into these and other theories, I want you to see this is exactly how the immune system and hormones and other systems in the body behave. It's a constant ebb and flow of yin and yang.

That's what a negative feedback loop is. Something gets too yin and yang intervenes, or visa versa.

How the Ancient Chinese Understood the Immune System

The way the ancient Chinese described immune function was by calling it wei qi. They described this "defensive substance" that flowed into the gut deep into lymphatic vessels, which also carry absorbed dietary fat and lymph fluid.

In the body, the lymphatic system drains into the venous blood supply at the subclavian vein. This is a large vein located just below your clavical., which is visible in the drawing that you saw at the top of this chapter. There is a description of this in the *Nei Jing Suwen*, or *Yellow Emperor's Classic,* a seminal classic of Chinese medicine from the second century BC.

"Defensive substances (wei qi) are the fierce and brave vital substances of water and grains. Defensive substances are high spirited, travel quickly, are smooth and sliding in nature, and are not directly absorbed into blood vessels. Thus, defensive substances flow between the skin and muscles (the superficial lymphatics), vaporize in the membranes, and spread or disperse in the chest and abdomen."

These were the first descriptions ever of the body's immune system (2000 years ago). They understood subtle details like the fact that this wei qi leaves arterial circulation to mount a protective reaction and that it has both yin and yang characteristics.

In other words, they described the process of something leaving the bloodstream to protect the body. And that it was both yin and substantial (the lymph fluid) and yang and energetic (it caused an energetic reaction or triggered other events – the way the immune system causes many different changes in other systems of the body).

In addition, they spoke of immune reactions in both yin and yang terms. The inflammatory reactions of the immune response are considered yang and the anti-inflammatory functions are yin. This truly expresses the contradictory nature of the immune system we described earlier. It's not linear. Different parts of the immune system do different things. Sometimes the same part does things in opposite directions. Yin and yang describe this behavior quite well.

In addition to normal immune functions, this wei qi also has a role in warming the body and controlling pores and sweating. Wei qi functions also include control over superficial vasodilation and the immune complement system.

Understanding the Complement System

The complement system is a group of small proteins that basically add lighter fluid to a fire. They get the killers and attackers in the immune system amped up and make the carnage much worse during an immune response. These are the guys we want to clear out because of their destructive potential.

One other interesting thing about the Chinese medical approach is that it looks at these internal organs and their connections, or spheres of influences.

It is like having friends, family, and acquaintances that you have some degree of influence on. Well, it is the same scenario with each element.

So the metal element has the lung and large intestine and has the wei qi that we just described. It has the skin, the mucous membranes, and the nose. Which endocrine gland is connected to it?

The thyroid. Holy crap! Just look at all the lymph glands in the throat. The thyroid is very much connected to the immune system.

And check this out. TSH is not only produced in the pituitary. Thirty years ago, it was discovered by researchers that immune cells actually produce TSH during times of acute infection.

Where do the immune cells produce TSH? They produce it in the bone marrow where immune cells are born, by white blood cells, and also in the intestines when exposed to a virus. Remember when we were talking about IL-18 and IL-12? Well, it turns out they also produce TSH.

Here's an Example

A female patient's lab tests said her TSH was too high, yet she was having many hyper symptoms such as anxiety, palpitations, mood swings, and so forth. She was going nuts.

Think about this. She had some gluten and dairy (made from cow's milk), which caused a massive immune response in her intestines. She may have been exposed to some sort of pathogen (maybe a bovine virus) and those immune cells produce TSH.

Her TSH appeared high because of these factors, but she was functionally hyperthyroid. Remember in an earlier chapter how I said what you feel is diagnostically and clinically important with Hashimoto's?

This can work both ways. A hypothyroid state creates impaired immune function. At this time, a lot is still not known about this, but one of the theories is that immune cells produce a local surge of T3, and this surge causes a systemic decline in TRH and TSH production.

One theory on this is that in times of infection and immune induced inflammation (which autoimmune disease is a chronic state of), the immune system shuts down thyroid function and then at some point kicks it back in again.

Well, with Hashimoto's, this endocrine-immune communication is out of whack. The immune system may not be able to kick things in again. Or it may not know when the "infection" is over due to chronic inflammation and tissue attack.

The antigen is the tissue of the body. The fight never stops. You understand what I'm saying?

To be honest, I just learned about this in researching this book. We are looking at some cutting edge stuff people! Wow. And 2,000 years ago these Chinese masters put this together.

Put that in your pipe and smoke it! (No, not good for your lungs, don't do that!)

The Emotions of the Metal Element

The *Nei Jing*, or *The Yellow Emperor's Classic of Medicine*, a classic text that dates back 2,200 years, describes the lungs as minister and chancellor. It helps the heart to regulate the body's qi or energy.

The lungs govern the wei qi, which guards our outer most boundary, and prevents all that doesn't match our true self from getting inside to our core. Grief is the negative emotion of the lung, and grief can weaken them.

My father died when I was nine. The next year I got pneumonia. Maybe it was a coincidence or maybe there is some connection.

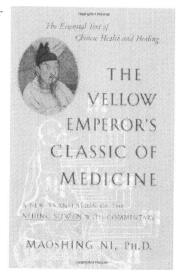

The lungs are very vulnerable to dryness, as well. If this boundary to self becomes too dry, then finding our true self can become more difficult. If the lungs become too moist, then phlegm builds up and blocks our connection to the essence of life.

In health the lungs are thought to empower us to stay connected to the essence of value even after the material things disappear. For example, after the loss of a loved one, a healthy lung can empower a connection to the spirit of that person.

But if the lung is weak, you could become fixated on the loss, become lost in that grief, and lose appreciation of the present moment.

This grief can become manifest as phlegm, a chronic cough, constant dripping sinus, like internal tears. Phlegm is a very important thing in Chinese medicine. Like qi, it has a number of different definitions.

Good phlegm clears pathogens; it's the first line of defense. Bad phlegm, ("Bad Phlegm!"), accumulates in the joints, the kidneys, the brain, and the thyroid in the form of nodules.

In the Chinese character of phlegm, we see the character that means inflammation. Phlegm can also represent the antibody response to pathogens that cross react to healthy tissues.

This kind of phlegm impairs cellular immune function leading to chronic disease.

Understanding the Large Intestine's Role

The large intestine is the yang partner to the lung. According to the *Nei Jing*, the large intestine is responsible for transit. All waste products go through this organ.

This is true of waste moving through the large intestine, which returns to the earth. It's also true metaphorically. The large intestine constructs a barrier between self and non-self by sorting out the things we take in and then determining which acquired influences need to be kept and which need to be let go.

With autoimmune disease, so much of which begins and is perpetuated in the intestines, the barrier between self and non-self, is lost. We lose self-tolerance. And a lot of this happens in the intestines.

Failing to respond in a balanced way to loss in life (and not just loss of a loved one—any loss: a job, a relationship, a pet), the large intestine reacts to the presence of grief and longing.

This grief can become distorted and it can be difficult to let go in that you keep holding on to things that no longer serve you. And what happens? Diarrhea—where you loose important minerals, or constipation where you are literally holding onto things that no longer serve you.

This condition can make you pessimistic, cynical, and generally negative. It can make you judgmental of others. Leaky gut or intestinal permeability is caused by a breakdown of the intestinal lining and cell walls.

Many researchers believe that it is one of the root causes of autoimmunity and the loss of self tolerance. (We will explore this in depth in the section on the Earth Element.)

Leaky gut may also have an emotional root. It can make you feel not properly valued by others. You see how this is all connected?

Let's now look at some important insights that Chinese medicine offers in the treatment of autoimmune disease in general and Hashimoto's in particular.

In the last chapter we talked a lot about normal lab tests and lots of symptoms. Well another thing that "bad" phlegm does is block receptor sites and impair thyroid hormone binding, which can affect the lab test results and also prevent thyroid hormone from working as well in the body.

Three Important Treatment Strategies

There are three important treatment strategies that can be employed by using Chinese herbs to treat autoimmune disease. All three processes that these strategies address are involved in the initiation and continuation of autoimmune disease. If we want to slow or stop the progression, we may have to deal with these pathogenic processes.

1. Deal with pathogens. Chinese medicine uses the term, xie qi, for these pathogenic influences. One of these pathogens is wind. There is wind cold, wind heat, and so on. Wind is a metaphor for airborne pathogens such as viruses, bacteria, and so forth. Entire schools of Chinese medicine are devoted to the treatment of epidemic diseases caused by these pathogens. Long before the invention of antibiotics and anti-virals the ancient Chinese treated these diseases with herbs.

In fact, when we look at the pharmacology of the herbs used to treat these conditions, they turn out to be broad spectrum antibacterial, antifungal, and antiviral. As we have seen, viruses like the Epstein Barr virus have been linked to Hashimoto's. Sometimes these viruses can linger for years and resurface. Other bacterial and fungal infections may also be present in the body and can undermine the healing process if they aren't dealt with.

2. Limit antibody cross reactions with healthy tissue. Cross reactivity is an important concept. There is an article about cross-reactive foods on our website in the supplemental materials as well.
https://hashimotos-diet.com/roadmap-to-remission-supplemental/

Here's the concept: All proteins, including viral proteins, are built from amino acids. In nature there are twenty different amino acids and they comprise the proteins of every living substance on earth.. Many are very similar in structure, and since your immune system attacks these proteins, sometimes immune cells may attack the wrong things because they resemble this protein structure.

Different antibodies then attack both tissues that look alike. For example, gluten resembles cerebellar tissue. Eat gluten, and immune cells may attack your brain. This is one theory why some autistic children may do better on a gluten-free diet. Researchers Brinmberg L., et al, found strong evidence that brain reactive antibodies were increased in mothers of children with autism.

Depending upon which antibodies and which tissue, we can choose herbs that focus on cross reactivity. There are even herbs that can be helpful for thyroid enlargement.

Other herbs are thyroid protective.

There are also other herbs that increase or decrease thyroid hormone, etc.

3. Slow or stop immune activation that is causing tissue destruction.
It is critically important to unwind this destructive process; well, you can actually clear circulating immune complexes with Chinese herbs.

Nothing in Western medicine does this except a very expensive process called, plasmaphoresis, where they essentially take out all your blood, clean it, and cycle it back in. You know, the Keith Richards treatment.

These immune complexes are amping up the attack. By clearing these you can really help calm down the immune system.

A list of those, too, are available in the next chapter. We have many of these herbs in our herbal pharmacy.

One Weird Herb that Has Superior Healing Properties

One herb, in particular, I'd like to highlight is Cordyceps. This is really an amazing herb and it is a fungus that grows on the bodies of silkworms.

Okay, time out! How'd they find this one? I imagine the conversation going something like this.

"Hey, what's that?"

"A silkworm."

"What's wrong with it?"

"What do you mean?"

"What's that all over it? It looks like mold."

"I don't know, let's eat it and find out."

Seriously? God bless the brave souls who had the courage to try and test these substances. Without them, we would never have discovered their amazing healing properties.

It actually has a kind of chocolaty taste. It also helps the body make glutathione.

The stuff is amazing. It is used traditionally to tonify kidney yang. Remember earlier we spoke about kidney yang being the source of endocrine function? It also tonifies the lung and dissolves phlegm.

Well, since it helps the body make and use glutathione, and glutathione has been shown to modulate immune function, wow and wow!

Pharmacologically, it's miraculous. Its antibiotic, anticancer, it relieves asthma, it stimulates immune function, it stimulates the adrenal glands, and it has been found to increase platelets.

All this from a fungus that grows on silk worms. Yum!

A Review of Chapter 5:

Okay, let's wrap up this section. So much has been covered. I mean mind-blowing stuff here, people! Let's recap.

1. The metal element in Chinese medicine has many components of the immune system. The lungs and large intestines are yin and yang pairs, and we can clearly see their connection through the lymphatic system. Wei qi is how the ancient Chinese explained the immune system and its activity.

2. Emotionally the lungs and large intestines help us deal with boundaries and loss. Grief is the negative emotion of the metal element. If the lungs are weak, you can get overwhelmed by grief and loss.

3. Phlegm is a byproduct of this process and in Chinese medicine phlegm is a pathogen, something that makes you sick. Bad phlegm can actually clog receptor sites and create nodules.

4. Chinese herbs can actually clear out circulating immune complexes, and Western medicine has no drug for that. These herbs can really help calm the immune attack. Specific herbs are also available for the various interleukins we talked about in this chapter.

5. Cordyceps, a fungus that grows on the bodies of silk worms is one example. Cordyceps helps clear out immune complexes that can increase the destructive attack by the immune system and it helps the body make glutathione.

Let's Appreciate Glutathione

I would like to take this opportunity to just heap praise on glutathione. The stuff is also amazing.

Glutathione is like the loyal bodyguard who will sacrifice his own life to save the life of the person he or she protects. There are different forms of glutathione in the body, but when we have enough of the right kind, we are protected from all kinds of toxic invaders.

However, when our glutathione stores start to run low, it triggers a destructive inflammatory process. Toxic chemicals and pollutants drain glutathione from the body because it is exactly what our bodies use to clean these destructive compounds out of our systems.

Glutathione is also everywhere. It's in animals, microorganisms and plants and, because it is water-soluble, it's found mainly inside cells. In fact, it is one of the most highly concentrated antioxidants inside of cells.

There are different forms of glutathione available on the market. It's important to know which kind does what. The oral form of S-Acetyl-L-Glutathione can be utilized by the body and is mostly absorbed by the liver. There are liposomal creams that are absorbed by the peripheral tissue and that are effective for getting it into the blood stream and into the thyroid, itself.

Then, there are other things, like cordyceps mentioned above, which helps the body recycle and reabsorb glutathione. Some doctors also offer it in IV form.

It is often depleted with Hashimoto's. It also strengthens (along with Vitamin D3) the regulatory or Th3 part of the immune system.

It does it all. I thank you, glutathione!

Chapter Eight

Using the A.P.A.R.T. System to Heal the Immune System

The A.P.A.R.T. System

1. A = Ask and Assess: An Overview of Immune Testing

Grab your journal and look for symptoms of problems with the Metal Element. Note what they are, then create a plan for addressing them. After that, you must act on your plan. Follow through and do what you have planned.

After that take inventory of what you did. Look at what worked and what didn't. Both will provide valuable information.

Double down on what worked, change what didn't. Keep refining your process.

Autumn is a good time of year to address Metal Element issues. (But don't wait to heal the intestines or lungs if something comes up at another time.)

Let's review a couple of things about testing and its availability for the immune system, particularly autoimmune disease testing and why it matters.

Signs and Symptoms of Autoimmunity and Barrier System Compromise:

Ask: Do you have any of these symptoms?

- **Lung Deficiencies**

- **Common Lung Disorders**

The Impact of Hashimoto's on the Lungs

The impact of Hashimoto's and hypothyroidism on the lungs and respiratory system is seldom discussed. However, there are a number of potential issues that may need to be addressed.

One thing we know is that fatigue and dyspnea (difficult or labored breathing) are common symptoms. These are some of the factors that make exercise such a challenge for Hashimoto's folks.

One explanation for this exercise intolerance could be the effects of hypothyroidism or "functional hypothyroidism" on the lungs, namely: limited pulmonary reserve, limited cardiac reserve and decreased muscle strength (especially of the diaphragm and other muscles involved in breathing).

Lower oxygen saturation has also been noted (this is interesting because when you combine this with the various anemias that are found in Hashimoto's patients, you have recipe for compounded fatigue).

Plueral effusion (or the build up of fluids in the interstitial spaces between the lungs and the tissues that line the chest) has also been found to be caused by hypothyroidism. One theory is that hypothyroidism leads to capillary permeability and fewer, narrower tiny vessels, as well.

In clinical practice, I have noted that complaints to the upper airway are common with people with Hashimoto's. Patients frequently complain of nasal congestion, recurrent colds, voice change, feeling of swelling or a foreign body in the throat, and discomfort and dryness of the throat.

Increases in nasal mucous may be increased, and about 20% of patients have tonsil enlargement. Sleep apnea is also found in this population and hypothyroidism is a well documented cause of obstructive sleep apnea. For all of the reasons mentioned above. This tends to be more severe in those people who are obese.

In addition to the issues that may be linked to hypothyroidism, many problems of the lungs (and large intestine) are due to a sedentary lifestyle that is also common in this day and age. Lack of activity can lead to poor respiration and elimination.

Lung and colon problems are, obviously, also made worse by a poor diet: overeating; not eating enough roughage; consuming too much dairy, sugar, processed foods, or other congesting foods. In addition, using recreational drugs, cigarettes, and pharmaceutical drugs, can also compromise lung function.

And Hashimoto's and hypothyroidism can lead to chronic constipation.

These habits and behaviors can cause mucus to be deposited into the lungs, which blocks their proper functioning. Colds, allergies, sinus problems, bronchitis, and asthma are some of the issues that may result.

Furthermore, toxins build up in the lungs and colon and create tension, exhaustion, hair loss and skin problems, like acne. The following syndromes give a sense of how these various conditions manifest in the lungs, and thus shed light on how to resolve them.

Common Syndromes of the Lungs

Viruses most commonly cause the first lung syndrome—the onset of conditions such as the common cold and flu. As we discussed, some viruses have also been linked to the onset of Hashimoto's.

(In the patient population I have seen, the Epstein Barr virus is the most common virus, and I've seen this in the history of more than 75 percent of the people I have spoken to and worked with.)

It is important to note that the practice of prescribing antibiotics for viral respiratory infections is not only a bad strategy but also has now been found to cause long-term damage to the immune system by killing off beneficial bacteria that are so important to healthy immune function.

In addition, overuse of antibiotics has now made us vulnerable to "super bugs" or drug resistant bacteria. Many effective herbal formulas are available that are quite effective for treating upper respiratory (sinus, ear, and lung infections).

If such infections are not resolved, they can develop into what is known as "heat in the lungs."

Heat Congestion in the lungs will usually have what are known as "exterior symptoms" in Chinese medicine, such as fevers accompanied by chills, and a red tongue with a dry, yellow coating.

In addition, dry cough, shortness of breath, and a painful sore throat may be present; there may also be thick, yellow-green phlegm, or even in more severe cases, blood streaked phlegm; and yellow nasal discharge.

It's important to have alternative approaches to healing these types of issues because when people with Hashimoto's become sick, it can be very debilitating.

Prescribing more and more antibiotics can further damage the ecosystem of the intestines. In some cases they may be necessary, but they should not be the first course of action, especially, if the issue is caused by a virus.

Treatment in Chinese medicine involves adding foods and herbs, which cool the heat and transform phlegm in the lungs. (See suggestions for these foods below).

Phlegm in the lungs is also most often brought about by weak digestion (weak spleen/pancreas) that causes mucus. It can also result from too much mucus forming food.

In either case, mucus accumulates in the lungs; symptoms include cough, shortness of breath, wheezing, or asthma accompanied by sticky phlegm. The tongue coating may be greasy and white if the phlegm is cold; a greasy yellow coating indicates hot phlegm.

Large Intestine/Immune Issues

Large Intestine Issues: Feeling that bowels do not empty completely, constipation, hard, dry, or small stool, frequent laxative use.

Intestinal Permeability Issues: Increased frequency of food reaction, unpredictable food reactions, aches, pains, and swelling throughout the body, unpredictable abdominal swelling, frequent bloating and distention after eating, abdominal intolerance to sugars and starches.

Chemical Intolerance: Multiple smell and chemical sensitivities, such as intolerance to smells, intolerance to jewelry, intolerance to shampoo, lotion, detergents, and constant skin outbreaks. (This is related to the Metal element because multiple sensitivities could be an indicator of a breakdown of the barrier systems. Both the lungs and intestines are 2 important barriers in the body).

Top 3 Foods That Can Lead to Autoimmune Flare Ups

From both my personal and clinical experience, I have found that the top three foods that may over-stimulate your immune system are gluten, dairy, and soy.

1. Gluten: Gluten is rich in lectins (Nature's own insecticides). It can bind to your intestinal walls, cause them to break down, and once through can cause a massive immune response.

Research also suggests that the proteins in gluten resemble certain tissues in our body. For example there is evidence to suggest that antibodies for gluten also attack Pukinje cells in the cerebellum. Threfore, when you eat gluten, your body attacks and attacks that tissue.

(We saw earlier in the chapter what a massive impact being on a strict, gluten-free diet can have.) More information concerning Hashimoto's and Celiac disease is found in later in this book and is available on our website in the supplemental section:
https://hashimotos-diet.com/roadmap-to-remission-supplemental/

2. Dairy: Dairy products are some of the most immuno-reactive substances in our diet. Commercial dairy is full of antibiotics and hormones, and the process of pasteurization leaves billions of dead bacteria and viruses. Raw dairy products have live bacteria and viruses. Raw, organic, grass fed may be tolerated, but is still a big risk.

And the issue with dairy is not what animal it comes from or whether or not it is raw or pasteurized. It is the problems caused by dairy proteins like casein and dairy sugars like lactose.

For an in depth discussion on Hashimoto's and dairy visit our website and read the supplemental materials:
https://hashimotos-diet.com/roadmap-to-remission-supplemental/

3. Soy: Soy is heavily genetically modified, is also rich in lectins, and is very difficult to digest. It is also estrogenic (it acts like estrogen) in large quantities. Soy can be anti-inflammatory, but can also be goitrogenic and suppresses TPO (not TPO antibodies). Okay, in small quantities if you can tolerate it, but many Hashimoto's people cannot.

In some people, these foods can cause massive broad spectrum immune responses.

Assess: Here are some tests you can do to find out more.

Low Tech and Lab Tests

Low tech tests are tests you can do at home. Lab tests, obviously, we order from the lab. Both can be helpful diagnostically.

Basically, low tech tests are challenge tests. They involve stimulating the immune system and seeing what happens. They can be risky and should not be done with certain types of people.

For example, if someone is very weak and depleted, stimulating the immune system could potentially wipe them out. So be cautious. That being said, they can also be really helpful.

Conceptually, whenever you eat something, whether its medication, herbs, vitamins or food, it has an impact on your immune system.

And if parts of your immune system are overactive and you take or eat something that stimulates that part of your system, then you can put gasoline on the fire and end up feeling like utter crap.

Does that make sense?

Th1 and Th2 Challenge Test

Natural remedies like herbs can cause more specific responses in the Th1 or Th2 systems. This can be helpful diagnostically; because it can help you identify things that may make you feel worse.

Basically, what you do is take a mixture of herbs that stimulate Th1 or Th2 and you do this for three days. Then you record your symptoms in your journal. You only take one of these at a time and you make sure that you limit other things that may be immune stimulating during this time. By minimizing the variables you can get a better sense of whether you are having a reaction.

(And this same methodology can be applied to everything in your life. Simplify, minimize the variables and test that particular herb, food or behavior and see how you react. And if they cause an immune response, it may be something you need to pay attention to and eliminate or avoid.)

When testing TH-1 and TH-2, lots of things can happen. You can get a reaction from one, or from both, or from neither. You need to keep a journal and note anything that is out of the ordinary.

If you get a reaction that could mean a flare up of your symptoms like pain, fatigue, brain fog, diarrhea, digestive complaints, and neurological symptoms like mood changes, anxiety or depression, etc.

And that is important because it can help you identify what to avoid. Sometimes these reactions are subtle so try and note anything out of the ordinary.

Here's a good list of TH-1 and TH-2 stimulating compounds that comes from Mickey Trescott, author of the Autoimmune Paleo Cookbook.

Th1 stimulating compounds:

Astragalus
Chlorella
Echinacea

Glycyrrhiza (found in licorice)
Grape Seed Extract
Medicinal Mushrooms (Maitake and Beta-Glucan are common)
Melissa Oficinalis (Lemon balm)
Panax Ginseng

Th2 stimulating compounds:

Caffeine
Curcumin (found in turmeric)
Genistin (found in soybeans)
Green Tea Extract
Lycopene (found in tomatoes and other red fruits excluding strawberries and cherries)
Pine Bark Extract
White Willow Bark
Resveratrol (found in grape skin, sprouted peanuts, and cocoa)
Pycnogenol (found in the extract of the French maritime pine bark and apples)
Resveratrol (found in grape skin, sprouted peanuts, and cocoa)
Quercitin (a flavanoid found in many fruits and vegetables, such as onions, berries and kale)

Don't Continue Once You Get a Reaction

And just to be clear, once you get a reaction. Stop. You don't need to keep causing a reaction and risk potentially hurting yourself. Note the reaction and stop.

Also, this type of test is not for everyone. For people who are very weak or people who have certain types of autoimmunity where a flare up can be life threatening, or for those people who are very compromised, this test can cause more harm than good.. You have to careful.

GABA Challenge for testing the Blood Brain Barrier

Another interesting challenge test is the GABA (gamma-aminobutyric acid) challenge. It can be used to test the blood brain barrier.

Why do we want to test this? Well, all the barriers in our body, the intestinal barrier, the lung barrier and the blood brain barrier are made of the made of the same proteins.

So if we find one to be compromised, there's a very good chance that the others are also damaged. We know that the gut and the brain have a very close connection. So if we find a weakened blood brain barrier, we know we have to intensify our efforts to heal the gut, as well. It's just a good, basic rule of thumb.

Because of the blood brain barrier and for other reasons; the immune system in the brain is much less specialized. It doesn't have all of the different immune cells and proteins and other forms of help we've been talking about.

Your brain has the microglia. And they are super hyper-vigilant. They're like paranoid chihuahuas with automatic rifles. They just start firing at the slightest sign of invasion.

This is why your brain reacts so strongly to immune stimulation. It just gets inflamed. And brain fog, memory issues, or concentration issues can also come from brain inflammation. One of the worst offenders? Gluten.

Regarding the GABA challenge, you simply take a large dose of GABA, 1000 mg., and you wait and see. Don't schedule anything important like driving heavy machinery or operating a chain saw for afterwards because you can end up with quite a buzz.

GABA is an inhibitory neurotransmitter. It calms things down. It can make you very mellow. But it's also a very big molecule and shouldn't be able to cross the blood brain barrier.

If you get buzzed, then you may have a breach. If you do have a breach, do not, under any circumstances, get chelation therapy until you've worked to heal that barrier.

(In an upcoming chapter we're going to get into the barriers and how to fix them.)

Chelation therapy draws heavy metals out of your tissues, and if you have a breach of the blood brain barrier, it could dump mercury, lead, cadmium, and other fun stuff right into your brain and other vital organs.

Very bad. Very, very bad. I've seen some patients who were never the same after chelation therapy. Seriously. There are consequences to doing different therapies.

This is another reason to be humbled and sensitive to the complexity and stakes involved with the body, in general and blood brain barrier, specifically.

The Best Test Is Your Own Body

All of these tests and the tests mentioned below can be very helpful, but the gold standard is the elimination diet that is the initial phase of the Autoimmune Paleo Diet. Like all tests, these tests aren't perfect and you may still have reactions to things that don't show up in testing.

Once again, the best way to test your body is to ask your body. First eliminate the food, herb or substance in question and then reintroduce it after a period of time (30 to 60 days). Make this food, herb or substance the only variable and then take note of the response(s) it gives you.

Responses can vary from digestive upset, pain, cramping, gas, diarrhea and/or constipation to neurological symptoms such as moodiness, anxiety, depression, brain fog, memory loss and other cognitive problems.

Laboratory Testing

The best lab that I have found for testing autoimmune related issues by far is called Cyrex labs.

Their tests are called arrays and they are extremely well designed and supported by an enormous amount of research.. They are great tools for identifying the triggers and for identifying what additional autoimmunity you may have.

This data allows us to make changes early and to stop or slow the progression of autoimmune disease to other parts of your body (where it can be very destructive and, in some cases, life threatening).

I think these are important enough to include here to give you a sense of how you or whoever you are working with can use these tests (called Arrays) and the data they provide to better design your treatment.

1. Array #2: Intestinal Antigen Permeability Screen

This array tests intestinal permeability or leaky gut. So many Hashimoto's folks have leaky gut, which can contribute to flare-ups because so much of the immune system is in the gut.

If this barrier is compromised, bacteria, viruses, protein fragments, yeast and other things that shouldn't be in the blood stream may get through and your immune system will never have a chance to calm down.

This becomes a constant source of immune flare up and this activation can drive the destruction of tissues in your body.

This blood test:

- Measures intestinal permeability to large molecules, which can inflame the immune system

- Identifies the damaging route through the intestinal barrier (between cells or through the cell itself)

2. Array # 3: Wheat Gluten Proteome Reactivity and Autoimmunity

Most doctors test two or three antibodies for gluten. This test looks at twenty-four different gluten antibodies so that you can:

- Accurately identify Gluten Reactivity

- Measure antibody production against nine wheat proteins and peptides and three essential structure enzymes

This is the preferred test for celiac disease and gluten sensitivity. This also may be a good test if you have a lot of neurological symptoms, such as brain fog, numbness, balance, or speech issues of unknown origin.

3. Array #4 Gluten Associated Cross Reactive Foods and Food Sensitivities

This is a great test if going gluten, dairy, and soy free isn't yielding results. Twenty-five other foods are known to behave like gluten and can cause an immune response. Here's how to find them quickly.

You could also do an elimination diet and then reintroduce these foods to challenge each of them.

- This test can help identify dietary proteins other than gluten that you may be reacting to.

- If a gluten free diet isn't getting you the results you had hoped for, this test may help explain why by identifying cross reactive foods.

4. Array #11: Chemical Immune Reactivity Screen

Array #11 tests for antibodies to environmental toxins. Here's the theory about what happens in your body with these toxins.

In today's world we are exposed to chemicals, heavy metals, pesticiceds and other toxic substances on a daily basis. When they enter your body, your immune system and your liver must try and get rid of them by neutralizing and excreting them.

During this process they may bind with your own proteins and create what's called a "neo-antigen," which is a hybrid of our own tissue and environmental toxins and that is what your immune system may attack.

This attack may cause a massive immune wind-up, and you get all the flare-up symptoms. These can have a big impact on the progression of this disease.

This test can tell you which chemicals are causing flare-ups so that they can be avoided. For some people this is an important piece of the puzzle.

5. Array #5 Multiple Autoimmune Reactivity Screen

This is the test that helps answer the question, "Where else is it?"

This test is also expensive, but the information is incredibly valuable as an early warning sign for where this disease may be progressing.

It looks at twenty-four different antibodies for autoimmune disease in places you never thought of: like your pancreas, your brain, your joints, your cell walls, and your stomach.

This can be an amazing tool for seeing the big picture and for understanding why certain treatments and strategies aren't working.

We know antibodies are predictive, so even if you don't have any symptoms related to a particular antibody, this information can be valuable for prevention and being proactive.

Array #5 is an incredible tool and may be recommended for those who need a little extra incentive to take the progression of autoimmunity more seriously. And fair warning, this can be a little scary, as well.

It would be a good idea to test the intestinal ecosystem for a variety of issues as well. You can read more about that in the next chapter.

6. Array #10: Multiple Food Reactivity Screen

Array #10 is a brand new test developed by Cyrex Laboratories, and it is a definite game changer.

It tests for 180 different "real world" antigens including cooked foods (because cooking changes their chemistry), raw foods, and food additives. By "real world" they mean actual chemicals and substances found in the food you are really eating.

These aren't antigens just developed in a laboratory. This test and Array #4 will give you a very complete overview of the problem foods in your diet.

The Large Intestine and "FODMAP"

FODMAP stands for a list of things that you would probably never say during a normal conversation: Fermentable Oligo-, Di-, and Mono-saccharides and Polyols. These different substances weren't connected before researchers found a common link between them (see below).

These are made from different kinds of sugars such as fructose, lactose, fructo- and galacto-oligosaccharides (fructans and galactans) and alcohols (also sugar) like sorbitol, mannitol, xylitol, and maltitol.

These all share 3 things in common:

1. They don't get absorbed very well in the small intestine. This can happen for many reasons, like a breakdown of the intestinal lining and a breakdown in the mechanisms that carry these particles across the intestinal barrier.

Also, brush border enzymes like amylase, cellulase and invertase may be depleted and other enzymes like hydrolases may be lacking, as well. And sometimes, it's just simply that these molecules are too big to cross the barrier and get absorbed.

2. They can also be small and "osmotically active" meaning they kind of grease the wheels and get things moving. One example is lactulose, which is a synthetic sugar that isn't digestable. In large enough doses it works like a laxative, making the stool looser and promoting faster movement through the bowels.

3. These substances tend to be fermented quickly by bacteria. The chain length of the carbohydrate determines how fast these sugars are fermented. The shorter the chain, the faster the fermentation.

Lots of Gas

All of this translates into lots of farting.

Yes, I said it, bad and often really stinky gas. Treating this condition involves removing these FODMAP foods from the diet. Google FODMAP diet and you will find a list of these foods.

2. P = Prioritize and Plan

Examine which issues are the most severe. This is, obviously, complicated and involves the intersection the immune system and the digestive system—where most of the immune system lives.

In my personal and professional experience, diet is the single most important thing in getting the immune system under control and in slowing and/or stopping the progression of autoimmune disease.

The diet we advocate is the Autoimmune Paleo Approach, also known as the autoimmune diet. We will explore this diet in depth in upcoming chapters.

3. A = Act and Adapt

Act and put your plan into motion. Then observe what the results are. Double down on what works and change what doesn't. And results should be apparent relatively quickly. If they aren't, you need to make changes.

Clincial Pearl: Another important thing to be conscious of when addressing the Metal Element and working with the immune system is that stimulating immune function can have some serious adverse effects.

As we have seen, stimulating parts of the immune system that are already over excited can make things significantly worse. Particularly if that part of your immune system is already attacking your own tissues (like your thyroid or your brain).

This is why the TH-1/TH-2 challenge test mentioned earlier can be helpful. But it's also important to remember this when you are treating other things like colds and flu. During these times you may forget and focus on trying to get better.

Common immune stimulants like echinacea, goldenseal and astragalus are all examples of herbs that might be recommended, but may not be such a good idea if you have Hashimoto's.

Instead a better approach may be to use herbal anti-viral herbs. One that I have used with good success is a popular patent formula of Chinese herbs called Gan Mao Ling.

This contains ilex root, evodia, chrysanthemum flower, vitex, isatis root and honeysuckle flower. It is useful as both preventative and after you've become sick to resolve it more quickly.

Metal: Dietary Solutions for the Lungs and Large Intestine

Foods for Common Metal Element Issues

Common Cold: Chinese medicine has categorized two types of cold related issues, *Wind Cold* and *Wind Heat*. They are considered two different conditions and have two different treatment approaches.

Wind Cold: This often occurs when there's a change in the weather and if you have a weak immune system. Symptoms include: chills, fever, no sweating, headache, body aches, and clear nasal discharge.

The best way to treat this is to try and sweat the pathogen out.

Foods to help aid sweating are: ginger, garlic, mustard greens, grapefruit peel, cilantro, parsnip, scallions, cinnamon, and basil.

Wind Heat: This is usually more serious and it has often progressed deeper into the body and may involve a more serious infection. Symptoms include: high fever, some chills, sweating, sore throat, cough, headache, body ache, and yellow or green nasal discharge.

Foods recommended are: Mint, cabbage, chrysanthemum flowers, burdock root, cilantro, dandelion, apples, pears, and bitter melon. In addition drink plenty of water and get lots of rest.

Foods to relieve Constipation: bananas, apples, figs, spinach, peaches, pears, pine nuts, sesame seeds, mulberries, grapefruit, yams, honey, apricot kernels, alfalfa sprouts, beets, cabbage, bok choy, cauliflower, and Chinese cabbage and salt water will help to move the bowels. (Epsom salts are commonly used as a laxative. Be very careful with this as this can have a pretty dramatic effect.)

Clinical pearl: Magnesium is also very helpful for treating constipation. There are a lot of different kinds on the market. Here's a brief breakdown of those best used for constipation, and other purposes.

Magnesium carbonate, which has antacid properties, contains about 45 percent magnesium.

Magnesium chloride / Magnesium lactate contain only 12 percent magnesium, but has better absorption than others, such as magnesium oxide, which contains five times more magnesium

Magnesium citrate is magnesium with citric acid, which has laxative properties.

Magnesium glycinate is a chelated form of magnesium that has some of the highest levels of absorption and it is an excellent choice for those who are trying to correct a deficiency.

Magnesium oxide is a non-chelated type of magnesium, bound to a fatty or organic acid. It has stool softening properties.

Magnesium sulfate / Magnesium hydroxide (milk of magnesia) are typically used as a laxative. Be aware that it's easy to take too much of these, so be cautious and use only as directed.

Magnesium taurate contains a combination of magnesium and taurine, an amino acid. Together, they tend to provide a calming effect on your body and mind

Magnesium threonate is a newer type of magnesium supplement that has shown promise due to its ability to get past the mitochondrial membrane inside of cells.

Great exercise for constipation:

A simple exercise for stimulating peristalsis (movement through the intestines) is to rub your belly clockwise 100 times.

Other Lung Related Issues

- **Treating heat congestion in lungs** : watercress, cantaloupe, apple, persimmon, peach, pear, strawberry, citrus, seaweeds, mushroom, daikon radish, radish, carrot, pumpkin, kuzu, cabbage, bok choy, cauliflower, chard, papaya, and white fungus

- **Treating phlegm in lungs: fennel,** fenugreek, watercress, garlic, other members of the onion family, horseradish, turnip, fresh ginger, daikon radish, mushroom, cereal grass, and seaweeds

- **Foods that specifically affect lungs and large intestine**: pungent foods—onion family, radish, especially garlic, turnip, ginger, horseradish, cabbage, daikon radish, and white peppercorn

- **Mucilaginous (create natural mucous) Foods**: seaweeds, chia seeds, and okra

- **Beta-carotene foods**: carrot, winter squash, pumpkin, broccoli, parsley, kale, turnip, mustard greens, watercress, wheat or barley grass, and common green, blue green and golden micro algea

Herbs for Modulating Immune Function

I. Here's a quick review of herbs that are TH-1 and TH-2 stimulants.

It is important to note that while there is a kind of yin and yang relationship that exists between TH-1 and TH-2, it's not always as simple as taking one to reduce the other. If someone is especially inflamed or reactive, it may be best to avoid both TH-1 and TH-2 stimulants to allow the immune system to calm down.

TH- 1 stimulating compounds:

Astragalus
Chlorella
Echinacea
Glycyrrhiza (found in licorice)
Grape Seed Extract
Medicinal Mushrooms (Maitake and Beta-Glucan are common)
Melissa Oficinalis (Lemon balm)
Panax Ginseng

TH-2 stimulating compounds:

Caffeine
Curcumin (found in turmeric)
Genistin (found in soybeans)
Green Tea Extract
Lycopene (found in tomatoes and other red fruits excluding strawberries and cherries)
Pine Bark Extract
White Willow Bark
Resveratrol (found in grape skin, sprouted peanuts, and cocoa)
Pycnogenol (found in the extract of the French maritime pine bark and apples)
Resveratrol (found in grape skin, sprouted peanuts, and cocoa)
Quercitin (a flavanoid found in many fruits and vegetables, such as onions, berries and kale)

II. Here's an overview of herbs that can increase or decrease various interleukins that we discussed above. These come from lecture notes Matt Van Benschotten, OMD, a brilliant herbalist and practitioner of

Chinese medicine. It is not recommended to take these herbs without the supervision of a skilled physician.

Due to the unpredictable nature of immune function, some herbs that may seem like a good idea may not be and those that may seem like a bad idea may actually be beneficial.

Some herbs may also exert apparently contradictory effects and impact both TH-1 and TH-2 pathways. Welcome to the immune system. ;)

As we stated earlier, test something as a single variable before you start taking lots of it. And don't just assume that it will have the same effect in your body as someone else's body.

1. TH-1 family cytokines.

A. IL-12 increasing: celosia, ginseng, lentinus, herbal formula Xiao Chai Hu Tang

B. IL-12 decreasing: eleuthrococcus, garlic, inula, salvia, herbal formula Ba Wei Di Huang Wan

C. IL-15 increasing: Herbal formula Si Jun Zi Tang: Bai zhu, fu ling, ginseng, licorice

TNF alpha decreasing: acorus, asparagus root, amellia, capillaris, cordyceps, fagopyrum, polygala, cooked rehmannia, smilax

TNF alpha increasing: achyranthes, aloe, coix, cordyceps, Reishi mushroom, ginseng, psedostellaria

2. TH-2 family cytokines.

A. IL-4 increasing: Agaricus mushroom, celosia, eleuthrococcus, fagopyrum, inula, perilla leaf, tripterygium

B. IL-4 decreasing: angelica sinensis, epimedium, garlic, polygala, pseudostellaria, Herbal formula: Liu wei di hung wan

C. IL-10 increasing: coix, garlic, heolen, inula, lentinus, Liu wei di huang wan.

D. IL-10 decreasing: cordyceps, perilla leaf, Xiao qing long tang

3. IL-1 family cytokines: It is recommended to avoid herbs that stimulate IL-1 and recommended to take herbs and supplements that decrease IL-1.

A. IL-1 decreasing: asparagus, lentinus, picrorhiza, polygala, cooked rehmannia, rhubarb, siegesbeckia, smilax, tinospora, turmeric, quercetin, bosallia, Clearvite formula

B. IL-1 increasing: achyranthes, Reishi mushroom, lentinus, American ginseng, tremella, typhonium

C. IL-18 increasing: lentinus, Ba wei di huang wan

III. Supplements for increasing TH-3, regulatory T cells: Vitamin D, EPA, DHA, glutathione, super oxide dismutase

IV. Supplements that decrease TH-17: According to Dr. Kharrazian the following substances reduce TH-17, largely due to their ability to increase healthy nitric oxide levels in the blood: Adenosine, Huperzine A, Vinpocetine, Alpha Glycerylphosphorylcholine (Alpha GPC), Xanthinol niacinate, L-Acetylcarnitine.

V. Herbs for Clearing Pathogens: These herbs have broad spectrum antibiotic, antifungal and anti-viral properties: chrysanthemum, cinnamon twig, coptis, dandelion, forsythia, houttuynia, lonicera, magnolia bark, rhubarb, scute, siler, stemona, dermatrol

VI. Herbs for Clearing Circulating Immune Complexes: angelica sinensis, atracylodes, bupleurum, cordyceps, persica, rehmannia, rhubarb, schizandra, Herbal formulas: Si Jun Zi Tang, Tao Hong Si Wu Tang

Qi Gong Exercise for the Metal Element
Reach for Happiness

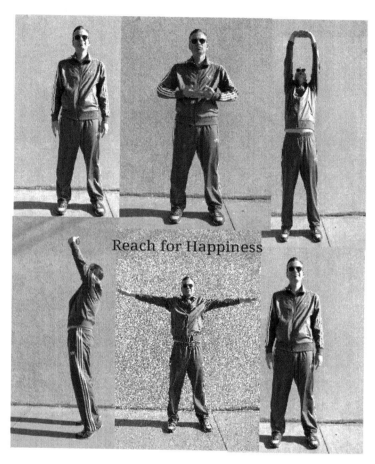

Reach for Happiness

This exercise focuses on bringing more energy and blood flow to the lungs. In Chinese medicine, the lungs are one of the most important organ systems for creating energy and sustaining health and well being.

This exercise has its origin in a famous statue of Bhudda in which he is portrayed with his hands above his head just like the photo above.

As we learned in the chapters on the Metal Element, the lungs and large intestines are untied by the immune system. And as you can see in this drawing they both have an enormous number of lymph glands in and around them.

So focusing on healing these areas can have a very positive effect on the immune system for calming, regulating, and balancing the immune system. All things that a valuable for people with Hashimoto's.

This exercise is also good for digestive problems; heart, lung, spine, or back problems; and a stiff neck and eye problems.

This exercise helps also bring more blood flow to the brain, increases lung volume, and increases blood flow back to the heart.

How to Do It: Begin with the natural standing posture. Feet shoulder length apart, hands hanging relaxed at yur side.

Inhale and gently sweep your hands out to your sides, to the front and bring your hands to meet at your abdomen, just below your navel.

Your palms should be facing up towards the sky, with your finger tips pointing up towards each other.As you sweep your hands up imagine that you are holding a ball of energy, keep your arms rounded and your armpits open.

Next raise your hands, lifting the energy ball slowly and steadily up to your chest. Keep your arms about 6 to 8 inches from your body to keep the movement open. Gently hold the energy ball and imagine that you must balance it or it will fall.

Next turn, turn the palms down and rotate your thumbs underneath and push your hands out above your head. Keep your fingers interlocking and again imagine that you are balancing an energy ball and pushing it far into the sky.

At the end of this movement stand up on your tip toes, as far as your balance allows. Push up for one or 2 seconds as you completely exhale. Then inhale as deeply as you can while staying relaxed.

Finally, exhale again, unlock your fingers and return your head and eyes to a forward position. Let your arms float outward as if gently pushing down a couple of big balloons.

Repeat the entire exercise 3 times, once or twice a day. When you are finished try to maintain the posture and height that got from doing the exercise.

Want to see a video demonstration of this exercise? Visit our supplemental page: https://hashimotos-diet.com/roadmap-to-remission-supplemental/

4. R= Reassess and Readjust

Retest, reassess and ask all over again. Figure out what worked and what didn't. Double down on what worked and either eliminate or recreate a plan for what didn't.

If you ordered diagnostic tests, reordering them will help you figure out if what you did changed anything. This can also get expensive.

You should also be keeping track of your symptoms and what you are doing in a journal. If you are doing this, you can often see patterns emerge. This can be very helpful for deciding what's working and what isn't.

Journaling and keeping track of your reaction to various foods, chemicals and other foreign substances can be really important when it comes to balancing and regulating the immune system.

If you continue to be exposed to things that your immune system reacts to and this is the same part of your immune system that is attacking your tissue, than this can become a problem that is never resolved.

5. T = Try and Try Again

Keep doing it, keep refining, keep building on the positive results, and keep looking for the remaining positive feedback loops that are causing vicious cycles.

This is a long term project. Play the long game. Keep at it and don't quit before the miracle.

In my experience this is where some people lose the will to keep going and they quit too soon.

Keep the faith, it will be rewarded.

Chapter Nine

The Earth Element:
Ground Zero for Autoimmunity

I am so excited to get into this chapter's topic, the Earth system, because this is really where it all happens with Hashimoto's.

The Earth system in Chinese medicine represents the digestive system.

The ancient Chinese identified this as being so important that there is an entire school of medical practice that was created around it called, appropriately, the Earth School.

Basically, they believe that almost every ailment comes from some problem in the digestive tract. And my experience with treating Hashimoto's folks has been the same. This is ground zero.

141

As you know, Hashimoto's is an autoimmune disease and a thyroid disorder.

And as we have explored in the first two chapters of this book, the digestive tract is a very important place for all aspects of this condition.

It impacts thyroid hormone and it is where most of the immune system lives. A healthy ecosystem in the gut is essential for converting and absorbing thyroid hormone and for balancing and calming immune function.

It's also hugely important for healthy brain function (which we'll cover in the chapters on the brain). What goes on in the digestive tract affects the whole family of ecosystems in your body.

Diet is the foundation of success

This is where it all happens, people. And if you don't work on your diet and healing the Earth element, you won't have success treating Hashimoto's.

It's just that simple.

If you doubt that this is true, a colleague and friend of mine, Dr. Izabella Wentz, recently shared the results of a survey she conducted with 2232 people with Hashimoto's.

On the question of diet, these were the results:

"In addition to the gluten-free diet, the other most helpful dietary interventions were going on a sugar free diet and the Paleo diet (81% of those who tried these diets felt better), grain-free diet (81% felt better), dairy free diet (79% felt better), autoimmune Paleo diet (75% felt better) and the low glycemic index diet (76% felt better)."

In this chapter we will discuss the reasons why these types of diets yield such good results.
However, before we jump into that, let's recap the important takeaways from what we've covered so far because these are related to what we're going to cover here.:

- We looked at thyroid hormone conversion and the role of good bacteria in converting T4 to T3, which the body can use. We're going to explore that a bit more in this chapter.

- We also looked at the Metal Element, which is the immune system. The lungs, the large intestines, the lymphatic system and, amazingly, the thyroid are all part of this.

- The lung and the large intestine are linked via the lymphatic system and represent our physical, emotional, and spiritual borders with the outside world and the boundary between self and non-self.

Remember, autoimmune disease is the loss of self tolerance and recovery, and healing of those borders and boundaries is an essential part of healing.

The Earth Element; Center of Healing

In some diagrams of the 5 elements, the Earth Element is pictured in the center and all the other organ systems surround it. In many ways, it is the center of healing.

The Earth element includes the spleen, stomach, pancreas, and the whole digestive tract. As we explore it in more depth, you will discover that is also the center of autoimmunity.

As we look at the Earth system, try to be open to the fact that we don't know everything and only through observation and questioning the status quo can we hope to learn.

There's something in psychology known as confirmation bias, this is the unconscious act of referencing only those theories and ideas that agree with our pre-existing views. This leads to ignoring other theories and ideas that may actually lead to breakthroughs and progress.

The Appendix is a Perfect Example

Did you hear the news that scientists think they have finally figured out what the appendix was for?

For many years the established dogma was that the appendix was an artifact, a useless piece of flesh that evolution somehow forgot and, therefore, could be simply removed, without the slightest repercussions.

Well, the truth is that nature is infinitely more clever than man and infinitely better at using everything that exists for some purpose. Nature does not forget things. If they have no purpose, they almost never survive evolution.

Well, so it is for the appendix. It turns out it has a purpose.

What is it?

The appendix is actually a bank of good bacteria, so that when there is a die-off, or a full frontal assault for whatever reason, it acts to replenish your intestines with the species that are beneficial.

The right bacteria are hugely important for many things. And one important thing with regard to Hashimoto's is the role of the gut bacteria to assist in converting inactive T4 into the active form of thyroid hormone, T3. As you learned in chapter 1, about 20 percent of T4 is converted to T3 in the GI tract.

Good bacteria helps convert thyroid hormone

Good Bacteria Helps Convert Thyroid Hormone

It is converted in the forms of T3 sulfate (T3S) and triiodothyroacetic acid (T3AC). The conversion of T3S and T3AC into active T3 requires an enzyme called intestinal sulfatase.

Where does intestinal sulfatase come from?

Drum roll.........

Yup, you guessed it, a healthy balance of bacteria in the ecosystem of the gut. When this ecosystem is out of balance and there are less benefical bacteria than other species, then this can affect the rate of conversion of T3S and T3AC to T3.

Here's where we see how events outside the thyroid can cause problems with thyroid hormone in the body. This is another factor that can lead to "functional hypothyroidism". Hypothyroid symptoms, but normal lab test results.

But established dogma said the appendix was an artifact and it had no purpose. And bacteria in the gut…hmmmm.

This is why things like observation and trying to figure out the mechanics are so helpful. When you can see what's going on, and find the mechanism, much becomes clear.

Nature always has a method to her madness. Man has dogma. Dogma says, "What I say is the absolute truth. Don't question it." Obviously, this can stop us from learning what the real truth might be.

Let's Talk Stomach

What does the stomach do and what is its relationship to the thyroid?

Well, it's role is to take food that has been chewed (hopefully, well) and mix it with saliva to break it down.

Okay, what breaks all this down?

Hydrochloric Acid

Hydrochloric acid is vitally important for breaking down vitamins, minerals (like iron), and vital nutrients so that they can be absorbed by your small intestine.

A lot of people, misled by dogma, think that stomach acid is bad. Two drugs in the top ten drugs prescribed in the US are Nexium and Prevacid. These medications are designed to block the production of stomach acid and are called proton pump inhibitors.

The proton pump inhibitors work by completely blocking the production of stomach acid. They do this by inhibiting (shutting down) a system in the stomach known as the proton pump.

This is another perfect example of sales and marketing trumping good clinical decisions. In 2013, according to Medscape.com, Nexium, alone totaled $6.1

billion dollars in sales. So this has led to the false theory that it's ok to suppress stomach acid, in some cases indefinitely.

There's only one problem: having enough stomach acid prevents food poisoning, parasites, and other critters from taking over your digestive tract. Enough hydrochloric acid also stimulates gall bladder and pancreas function to complete digestion and keep the entire digestive tract working properly.

Proton pump inhibitors also affect thyroid hormone absorption, and a study from *Endocrinology Practice*, the official journal of the Endocrine Society of America, found their impact so significant that patients taking these drugs and thyroid hormone may need to adjust their dosage.

So, you actually do need hydrochloric acid, or HCL, and its production depends on the hormone gastrin. And guess what has an impact on gastrin? Thyroid hormone.

So hypothyroidism causes less gastrin to be produced, which leads to lower amounts of hydrochloric acid, which in turn leads to heartburn, bloating, gas, . . .wait!

Did you say heartburn? Why, yes I did.

But didn't you also say too little hydrochloric acid? Why, yes I did. Ah hah! Gotcha.

Let me explain . . . mechanisms, people.

It turns out; having enough stomach acid actually prevents heartburn by thoroughly digesting your food. The burning sensation that people feel from heartburn is actually from the poorly digested food rotting in your gut and pushing up into your esophagus. This creates a kind of traffic jam.

And the esophagus has no protection from the acid. Even a small amount of can cause problems and irritation there.

In an editorial published in the *Journal Gastroenterology*, June 1, 2009, the author remarked:

"Treating gastroesophageal reflux disease with profound acid inhibition (which is exactly what proton pump inhibitors do) will never be ideal because acid secretion is not the primary underlying defect."

This is true.

For decades the medical establishment has been focusing on how to reduce stomach acid secretion in people suffering from heartburn and GERD.

Even though it's common knowledge that these conditions are not caused by too much stomach acid.

In fact, the real problem is too little stomach acid. So these drugs are insuring that the people who use them must continue to use them, indefinitely.

How Else Is HCL Beneficial?

Another thing that HCL is important for is the absorption of vital nutrients like B12, iron, and calcium, and for breaking down and absorbing protein.

Too little HCL can also lead to inflammation, lesions, and infections in the intestines.

All of that leads to poor absorption of thyroid hormone, which leads to... (This one is a gimmee)...*normal lab tests but hypothyroid symptoms and functional hypothyroidism.*

Too little stomach acid can also lead to anemia because you can't absorb B12, and you can't properly absorb iron.

Couple this with heavy bleeding during your cycle, which can also be caused by too little thyroid hormone and you have a recipe for iron deficiency anemia.

Wow, dogma, mechanisms, and the rantings of an addled Hashimoto's patient (that would be me).

Recap: Summary of Stomach

The stomach is important for breaking down and digesting foods, and for enabling the body to absorb important vitamins, minerals, and protein.

Too little stomach acid can lead to a host of problems: like heartburn (counter-intuitive but true), anemia, iron, and protein deficiency.

All of this creates a vicious cycle of less conversion and utilization of thyroid hormone and lower stomach acid. Not good.

In my clinical experience this is a very common, but under rated finding. Fixing this problem can make a really big difference because this affects everything downstream (i.e., the pancreas, the gall bladder, the intestines, etc.)

Now, let's go downstream, a bit and look at the pancreas and blood sugar issues.

Two Different Types of Sugar Problems

Health is really all about balance. And nowhere is this idea more evident than when you look at blood sugar balance.

There are really 2 different kinds of blood sugar problems and many people have a mixture of both. **These are hypoglycemia (or too little sugar in the blood) and insulin resistance (or too much sugar in the blood).**

With Hashimoto's either one or both of these blood sugar problems can make your symptoms worse. And just to remind you that this goes in both directions; it's important to understand that hypothyroidism can also cause blood sugar problems all by itself.

(We have the makings of a vicious cycle.)

Hypoglycemia

For your body low blood sugar is a really big deal. We are genetically programmed to react to low blood sugar because our lives literally depend on it. If we have severely low blood sugar or it continues for a long time our body can seize up, go into a coma or , worse case scenario, we could die.

When your blood sugar levels drop below normal, your adrenal glands answer the call by secreting cortisol. Cortisol then tells the liver to make more glucose, and the liver responds and brings blood sugar levels back to where they should be.

Hypoglycemia is a condition in which there is not enough cortisol to tell the liver to raise blood sugar into the normal range.

This process repeated day after day can end up wearing out the adrenals over time. In fact, we often see adrenal fatigue and hypoglycemia together. And

148

when you add the physiological stress of having an autoimmune disease like Hashimoto's, you have a recipe for both.

Low Blood Sugar and Cortisol

Cortisol is the body's fixer. It increases the amount of glucose available to the brain, and it helps speed up healing and tissue repair.

It also slows down functions that we don't need when we are in the middle of a crisis and our focus is to fight or run. Things like reproduction, growth and digestion. You can't eat, have sex and grow when you're in the middle of running for your life.

Having Hashimoto's is like living in a constant state of stress. Having autoimmunity is very stressful for your body and your brain. And this can lead to repeated cortisol release.

When you add this to low blood sugar, this can result in suppressed pituitary function. And the pituitary is the master gland that instructs the thyroid.

If this function isn't working properly, then "Houston, we have a problem." And where do we have a problem? In the thyroid.

Low Blood Sugar Causes Thyroid Problems

Cortisol directly inhibits the enzyme (5'-deiodinase) which converts inactive T4 into active T3. This can lead to low T3 levels.

In addition, elevated cortisol will cause thyroid hormone receptor insensitivity meaning that even if T3 levels are high enough, they may not be able to bind normally to receptor sites. And when this happens it doesn't get into the cells.

Cortisol will also increase the production of reverse T3 (rT3) which is inactive. (It's kind of like the anti-hormone.)

rT3 can cause an increase in the production of substances known as thyronamines that can cause hypothyroid symptoms (like, low basal body temperature,fatigue, depression, etc.) along with insulin resistance symptoms of increased blood sugar.

Cortisol can also lower the levels of protein that binds to thyroid hormone so it can circulate in a stable structure.

And finally, elevated cortisol will slow TSH production by disrupting hypothalamic-pituitary feedback leading to lower TSH production.

Well, there is also an HPT (hypothalmus-pituitary-thyroid) axis.
And much like wires going through a transformer on an electric grid, the HPT and HPA axis are very closely related and problems in one area can affect the other.

"When things go wrong, wrong with you, it hurts me too." sings the HPA to the HPT axis.

Common Symptoms of Hypoglycemia

Common symptoms of hypoglycemia include

(Many of these symptoms improve when you eat)

*Craving sweets
*Irritable if meals are missed
*Depend on coffee or other kinds of caffeine for energy
*Eating relives fatigue
*Feel shaky, or jittery
*Feel agitated or nervous
*Get upset easily
*Poor memory, forgetful
*Blurred vision

It's important for hypoglycemics to eat often throughout the day and not skip meals. Each meal should be a combination of protein, carbohydrates and fats. And, for these people, too many carbs will often cause serious problems with their blood sugar levels.

Insulin Resistance

When you eat too many carbs and too much sugar, the pancreas secretes insulin to move extra glucose from the blood into the cells where glucose is used to produce energy.

But over time, the cells lose the ability to respond to insulin. It's like insulin is a little dog barking outside the cell, but the cell won't let it in.

"I hear you barking, but you can't come in."

The pancreas responds by releasing even more insulin (barking louder) in an effort to get glucose into the cells, and this eventually causes insulin resistance.

Studies have shown that these repeated insulin spikes that come with insulin resistance increase the destruction of the thyroid gland in people with autoimmune thyroid disease (Hashimoto's).

As the thyroid gland is destroyed, what happens? Thyroid hormone production falls. And this causes hypothyroidism. Not good.

Insulin Resistance Can Lead to Thyroid Problems

Insulin resistance can also cause a reduced conversion of T4 to T3 hormones.

When this is addressed, the cells can once again start using glucose for energy and T3 production picks up.

So for a person who is insulin resistant, a lower carbohydrate diet may help restore better T4 to T3 conversion and often these people lose weight in the process (a nice side effect).

For other people, other things like long-term chronic stress may be affecting their response to low carb diets. Chronic stress can interfere with thyroid hormones in many different ways (we will explore these in the chapters on the Water Element).

Common Symptoms of Insulin Resistance:

(Eating generally doesn't improve these symptoms)

* **Fatigue after meals (this is the hallmark symptom)**
* **General fatigue**
* **Constant hunger**
* **Craving for sweets that isn't relieved when you eat sweets**
* **Must have sweets after meals**
* **Waist girth equal to or larger than hip girth**
* **Frequent urination**
* **Increased appetite and thirst**
* **Difficulty losing weight**
* **Migrating aches and pains**

Many People Have Symptoms of Both

Life is not a textbook. Many people are somewhere in the middle of this blood sugar odyssey and they have some symptoms of hypoglycemia and some symptoms of insulin resistance.

I put this question to my Facebook Support Group and of the 66 respondents with Hashimoto's, 24 reported symptoms of hypoglycemia and 14 reported symptoms of insulin resistance. 16 reported some symptoms of both. In addition, in the patient population I have treated I have found about 80% have symptoms of hypoglycemia, insulin resistance or both.

While this is hardly a scientific study, it does demonstrate how common this problem is in this population.

Virtually Everyone Has Some Insulin Resistance

On thing that's important to understand is that whether you have high or low blood sugar, you probably have some amount of insulin resistance.

I explained how high blood sugar causes insulin resistance above, but insulin resistance can also cause low blood sugar.

This condition, called reactive hypoglycemia, happens when the body secretes excess insulin in response to a high sugar and carbohydrate meal.

For example: A burger on a sesame seed bun, french fries and a soda – causing blood sugar levels to spike and then drop below normal. (I'm not lovin' it!)

Hypothyroidism Can Cause Blood Sugar Problems Too

If you eat like this and you have Hashimoto's (and hypothyroidism), you are setting yourself up for a world of hurt.

Hypo-function of the thyroid can cause everything we just talked about because:

- **it slows the rate that cells take in glucose;**
- **it decreases rate that the gut absorbs glucose;**
- **it slows response of insulin to higher blood sugar levels; and,**
- **it slows the removal of insulin from the blood by the liver.**

These mechanisms all appear clinically like hypoglycemia. When you're hypothyroid, your cells aren't very sensitive to glucose (they are resistant).

So although you may have normal levels of glucose in your blood, you'll have the symptoms of hypoglycemia (fatigue, headache, hunger, irritability, etc.).

And since your cells aren't getting the glucose they need, your adrenals will release cortisol to increase the amount of glucose available to them.

This causes a chronic stress response that suppresses thyroid function.

Does this sound familiar?

We've already discussed how some people are "functionally hypothyroid". In other words, they have enough thyroid hormone, but it's not getting into the cells.

Many of these people also have enough sugar in their blood but its not getting into the cells. It's another vicious cycle.

And let me tell you this from clinical experience. It is really, really, really, really, really, really, really, hard to manage a Hashimoto's patient or someone with functional hypothyroidism if he or she doesn't address their sugar issues.

In fact, I'm going to say it. It's a deal breaker.

If this high sugar diet or hypoglycemic state isn't treated, you might as well throw in the towel, pack it in, wave the white flag, say "Uncle", hear the fat lady sing, and give up, because it's just an exercise in futility.

All the money you're spending on supplements and therapies won't work. This is one of those areas that can undermine everything. That 20% that's causing 80% of your symptoms.

Keeping Blood Sugar in A Healthy Range

When balancing blood sugar, there are two things to consider. The first is fasting blood glucose, which can be measured first thing in the morning before eating or drinking anything.

The second, and more important thing to measure is post-prandial blood glucose. This is measured 1-2 hours after a meal.

In the final chapter of this section, we apply the A.P.A.R.T. System to the Earth Element, I have included a detailed description on balancing blood sugar using a glucose meter.

In conclusion, if you have Hashimoto's, it's also important that you take steps to make sure your thyroid is properly balanced to keep your blood sugar properly balanced.

As you have seen, this thing works in both directions.

Sugar problems can disrupt thyroid function, and thyroid disorders like Hashimoto's can cause sugar problems and put you at greater risk for hypoglycemia, insulin resistance and if nothing is corrected, diabetes.

This is why so many people feel better on a low sugar, low carbohydrate or Paleo diet. It is an excellent approach to fixing this blood sugar dilemna.

Recap: Blood Sugar Issues

1. Too much sugar in the diet leads to insulin resistance, and this can directly lead to more aggressive destruction of the thyroid in Hashimoto's.

2. Low blood sugar, or hypoglycemia, when it becomes chronic leads to cortisol release that eventually causes pituitary problems, which messes with thyroid function.

3. Hashimoto's and hypothyroidism itself can lead to either one or both of these problems creating a vicious cycle.

4. If you don't take your blood sugar issues seriously, you will have tremendous difficulty getting your Hashimoto's under control.

HASHIMOMENT:
THE FUTILITY OF
WORRY

The negative emotion of the Earth element is worry.

With Hashimoto's, sometimes it seems like there's a whole lot to worry about.

It can be overwhelming trying to figure everything out.
And because we have to be our own health advocates, we have a lot on our shoulders.
And if you're like most people, you also have a family to take care of.
And all of these demands may make you feel like you can't get to what you need to do to feel better.

So you worry.

The problem with worry is that it doesn't help, at all. It just builds on itself and gives you more to worry about. And it can become self-fulfilling.

So a better thing to do is to stop, look around, and find things to be grateful for. When you're grateful, it leads to acceptance.

When you can accept, then things are less overwhelming.

And when you can find gratitude in adversity, you become more resilient.

So stop, take five minutes, and think about everything you are grateful for. Don't leave anything out. You can be grateful for even the most seemingly insignificant things. The flowers, the leaves, the air you breathe, the water you drink, your clothes, the roof over your head, your dog or cat, anything and everything.

Try it and share the results with us on our Facebook page: www.facebook.com/hashimotoshealing

Chapter Ten

The Chinese Medicine View
of the Earth Element

Let's take a look at the Chinese medical view of the Earth element. In Chinese medicine, the yang element of the Earth is the stomach, and the yin element is the spleen.

In previous chapters, when I discussed some of the theories of Chinese medicine, I mentioned how each of the five elements is the organ system and its sphere of influence.

The point I was making was that the emphasis of anatomy and physiology for the ancient Chinese was how those organ systems function. That was the first functional medicine.

How does it differ from Western medicine?

Well, Western medicine anatomy and physiology is often focused on distinct parts and their independent and distinct roles. Most specialists stay in their focus area and do not leave it to look at the larger picture.

They name conditions and diseases and try to fit a patient's signs and symptoms into the disease or condition that has been identified. Then they prescribe a drug protocol that has been designed to treat that disease or condition.

In Chinese medicine, the focus is on patterns of function, or dysfunction, and they pay a lot more attention to how a given disease or condition impacts the rest of the body. Additionally, they determine where it is in its progression.

Chinese medicine has theories for stages of disease. The name of the disease is far less important than the extent to which it has impacted the body and which organ system or systems have been impacted.

And the further a disease or condition has progressed, the more serious it is and, consequently, the more difficult it is to resolve.

The Longer You Wait the Harder Treatment Becomes

In fact, the Chinese have an old adage that goes something like this: "Treating disease after it is formed is like digging a well after you've become thirsty." And we can add to that: "the thirstier you are, the harder it is to dig the well."

I believe that thinking this way is very important when we look at Hashimoto's because it is precisely why I say that everyone's Hashimoto's is a little bit different.

No two people are at the same stage of development in this condition, no two people have the same level of involvement of the other organ systems, and no two people have the same life factors involved, such as genetics, stress, or diet.

These considerations become incredibly important, as we try to unwind the mess that Hashimoto's has created in your body.

And this is exactly why no cookie-cutter approach with a one-size-fits-all solution will work for Hashimoto's. We see this all the time: thyroid replacement hormone doesn't work for a lot of people; the (fill in the blank) protocol doesn't work for a lot of people, and so on.

In many cases, the best protocol is the one that takes into account all the different systems of your body that are impacted. And simply because this is so complex and can involved so many different parts of the body, it is virtually impossible to mass produce. And often, this requires doing a whole lot more than simply treating the thyroid.

I think by now, as you're less than half way through this book, you are starting to understand the complexity of Hashimoto's and how it is a multisystem condition that requires a multisystem approach to heal it.

The Spleen/Pancreas: It's a Hybrid

Okay, so now let's take a look at the Earth element and its sphere of influence. As I said, the yin organ is the spleen, and the yang organ is the stomach.

The endocrine gland associated with the Earth element is the pancreas. In fact, a lot of what the ancient Chinese ascribed to the spleen sounds, in my opinion, very much like the pancreas.

The other parts of the system that represent the Earth element are the mouth, saliva, flesh, or muscles. It governs the sense of taste.

The spleen governs digestion and keeps the blood circulating. We know that it is also responsible for cleaning old and dead red blood cells from the bloodstream. It also stores platelets that aid in clotting and coagulation.

The ancient Chinese recognized the spleen as an important organ for immune function. We know now that it also stores monocytes—the Pacman white blood cells—and that B and T cells are made and mature in the spleen.

Remember in the last chapter when we spoke about certain immune cells producing TSH? Well, some of those cells come from the spleen.

The sense organ associated with the spleen is the mouth and health issues involving the spleen sometimes manifest on the lips and the corners of the mouth.

The negative emotion of the spleen is worry or obsessive thinking, and the energy or vitality of the Earth element is intent.

This energy is linked with mental and physical activity of the body. Lack of desire or difficulty with coordination and movement of the body may reveal an issue with intent and therefore, the spleen.

This difficulty with coordination is a problem with moving and articulating the limbs, and it is associated with poor utilization of nutrients by the muscles.

What are they talking about? It could be insulin utilization—the state of insulin resistance that we spoke about in the last chapter.

Almost all cells in the body have insulin receptors. So intent involves a major mental component and is also under the influence of insulin, but not always for the purpose of just utilizing glucose. Insulin can also help with the uptake of certain amino acids.

Serotonin Is a Great Example

One interesting example of this relationship involves serotonin.

The brain's ability to absorb serotonin is enhanced by insulin. If you become insulin resistant, what happens emotionally? You lose this intent, you become depressed, and you crave carbs to try and make you feel better.

Do you see how this is all connected? These are examples of spheres of influence.

In a spiritual sense, this intent affects the digestive functions of thought that allows for the processing and assimilation of our life experiences in a nourishing way.

Unbalanced function leads to brooding, worry, and excessive thought patterns, such as obsessive compulsive disorders. People who think obsessively can become stuck in a pattern of thinking for thinking's sake alone and they don't get nourished by their experiences because they can't move on.

One of the health issues that is problematic for the spleen is dampness. Internally, this can take the form of phlegm. Phlegm is made in the spleen and then sent up to the lung.

Metaphorically, dampness is an accumulation of everything that should be nourishing, but instead has become a burden. In a psychological sense, it manifests as lethargy, boredom, mental sluggishness, obsessive thinking, and brooding.

On a physical level, phlegm dampness accumulates in the spleen, stomach, lungs, and large intestines. Sweetness is the flavor of the Earth element. We've seen the problems excess sugar can cause.

Well, from a spiritual/psychological standpoint, this phlegm dampness represents the excessive need to give or receive sympathy. Therefore, it's spiritual phlegm. It is giving too much and not taking care of yourself, or demanding too much so that it becomes a burden to others.

The Earth Has Always Been There for Us

The positive attributes of the Earth element are integrity and reciprocity or giving back equally. Integrity is being faithful and truthful. The sage or enlightened being is a person who is kind to the kind and to the unkind. He or she trusts the trustworthy and the dishonest, meaning he or she trusts nature.

The idea of reciprocity is really that of giving back appropriately what has been given to you. The Earth nourishes all of us; our planet is the ultimate in faith, trustworthiness, and loyalty. The Earth has always been here for us, for billions of years it has sustained life.

Well, we need to reciprocate and be good stewards of our planet or we're not going to survive as a species. Because, really when it comes down to it, what's happening to our world is also happening to our bodies.

Some feel that the rise of autoimmune disease may be a direct consequence of our larger inability to care for the Earth.

All the pollution, radiation, and global impact of man and industrialization is resulting in an environment that is becoming increasingly less supportive of good health.

Everything is connected; all the different ecosystems inside our bodies and all the ecosystems in our environment.

Of course, this is more philosophy than science. But what if we all behaved with that in mind?

Healing ourselves and healing the Earth would become synonymous.

Quick Recap

1. The Earth element is the spleen, stomach, and pancreas. The spleen is yin; the stomach is yang. The pancreas is the endocrine gland associated with the Earth element.

2. The negative emotion of the spleen is worry or obsessive thinking. This is linked to sugar metabolism and insulin resistance. We could see that the emotional consequences of insulin resistance can be depression, obsessive thinking, or emotional phlegm.

3. The positive attributes of the Earth element are integrity and reciprocity. It means being faithful and truthful and giving back to the Earth that has served us and given us life for billions of years.

It's All Connected

Isn't it amazing how all these things are connected? These connections are the fulcrums of healing; they are the places where we can get the best results. They are also our source of hope for healing our Hashimoto's.

Now let's look at the stomach in TCM terms.

In the *Nei Jing*, the Yellow Emperor's Classic of Medicine, the spleen and stomach's functions are mentioned together.

So that's interesting. And if we factor the pancreas into this equation, it makes sense. The functions of the stomach and pancreas are very much intertwined.

These two organ systems are really all about acquiring and distributing the nourishment of life.

The virtues of the earth element, integrity and giving back, can be seen in the stomach in the gathering and processing of all resources that are available in the outside world.

The spleen's job is to integrate what the stomach has acquired. And it does this by adding nutrients and building our blood. Through the blood, the spleen takes this information and distributes it to all aspects of our inner being.

The spleen makes this integrity live in us by incorporating the things that are part of our lives that are sympathetic to our inner being.

Another way to think of this is that it is the process of how we integrate the energies of heaven and earth into our own beings.

When you have a separation of mind and body, this sympathy can block the stomach from looking inward to the spleen to get a true sense of what we really need in life.

Then we seek poor sources of nourishment that are ultimately unfulfilling, like junk food pumped full of salt, fat, and sugar. This leads to obsessive behavior; you reject what is good for you or you over eat in an effort to just pile it on.

A Healthy Earth Element Means Healthy Boundaries

The Earth element impacts personal boundaries. It gets harder to distinguish between your needs and the needs of others. The breakdown of this boundary leads you to either be too needy of other people or to take care of other people too much, at your own expense.

If someone is too needy they become like a sponge, soaking up the emotional phlegm. They become too sweet, ingratiating themselves and sometimes manipulating others when they do this.

The other side of this Earth impulse is to look for intimate relationships with other needy or sick people so that you can put your energy into nourishing them back to health instead of nourishing and healing yourself.

163

We all have some of this. I had to identify this in myself and completely rethink my medical practice because I was doing way too much and I ended up losing my health as a result.

What are we trying to do in those circumstances?

Ultimately, we seek to care for others in the way that we wish we were cared for. But this can exhaust us and leave us depleted.

And what happens?

If you do a good job helping that other person, they don't need you any more. Then, if you are out of balance, you can get resentful that they don't appreciate you enough. You see this with a lot of healers; they give too much and get burned out.

First Heal Yourself, Then Help Others

So, to heal the Earth element, we must first heal ourselves and then when we help others we have the capacity to do it in a way that has integrity and balance.

It's just like being on an airplane. Put the oxygen mask on yourself first, then you can breathe and help other people around you.

How do we address these deep-seated emotional Earth Element challenges? Let's think about that. We have to nourish ourselves appropriately on this journey.

We have to transform this sugar burning/sugar binging mentality into one that is more integrated and ultimately more sustainable.

Does that make sense?

I'll bet you never thought that healing your Hashimoto's would mean actually healing your life too. Well, that's the journey.

We are in this for the long haul so that we can come out the other side and not only heal ourselves but also heal our relationships with one another and with our planet.

And, the truth is, if you don't address the dietary issues that are at the foundation of this process, all the herbs and supplements in the world won't give you the results you are looking for.

164

Quick Recap

1. I think we can see how the choices we make can have a huge impact on our lives. Especially with Hashimoto's, if you don't fix your blood sugar problems, you can't heal.

2. Well, this is also true on an emotional and psychological level. We have to heal the Earth element so that we can make appropriate decisions as to how much to give to others and how much to nourish ourselves.

3. We have to have balance, so that we can be faithful and truthful, yet be able to give to others without over giving and leaving ourselves malnourished.

4. We must also learn how to get proper nourishment so we don't become burdensome to others and so that we don't help others at our own expense, leaving us feeling resentful and unappreciated.

5. The foundation we use for healing is the Elimination diet and the Autoimmune Paleo diet. It can help heal your leaky gut, and it can heal and rebalance blood sugar imbalances.

And if we can do those things, then we've gone a long way towards healing the Earth element and getting our Hashimoto's under control.

It is by no means the only thing we have to fix, but it is sure taking some huge steps in the right direction!

Here's a real life story about someone whose Earth element was at the root of her issues.

This patient is a 45-year-old female who suffered from a history of serious gastrointestinal problems. (Used with permission)

A motility test revealed that her stomach wasn't emptying, she suffered from too little stomach acid (hypochlorydria), chronic constipation, bacterial overgrowth of the small intestines, and chronic yeast infections.

She could not digest fatty foods well because she had her gall bladder removed due to complications from the problems mentioned above. She also experienced fatigue after meals, which was extreme at times.

Unfortunately, and not surprisingly, she had a number of symptoms of intestinal permeability (leaky gut) and had difficulty maintaining proper iron levels along with other important nutrients, and she experienced vacillations in how her thyroid medication worked.

Sometimes she would feel hyper, and sometimes she would feel hypo.

Clearly this was a person whose Earth element needed some tender loving care. And that's just what we did.

We got her on a strict Autoimmune Paleo Diet, got her off of the foods that were causing more problems in her gut, and we worked on supporting detoxification in her liver and in healing her intestinal lining using supplements like brush border enzymes.

We also worked to rebalance and repopulate the ecosystem of her intestines.

After a couple of months of faithfully following our protocol, here is an e-mail we received from her:

This was a tremendous victory for her. Getting her serum iron into normal range "...for the first time in my adult life..." may not seem like a big deal.

But, in terms of energy, quality of life, and healing, this is a major achievement, and it allowed her to get her life back. She deserves the credit because she stuck with our plan and didn't whine or complain about not being able to eat certain foods.

She was in enough pain and discomfort where that hardly mattered any more. Now she is enjoying life in ways she had only dreamt about before.

Chapter Eleven

Leaky Gut or Intestinal Permeability & Other Issues

Breakdown of the intestines can happen between cells, through cells, or both.

I wanted to go into a little more detail on leaky gut in this chapter and also explore some additional obstacles you may encounter in your healing process.

First of all, what is leaky gut, and how does it lead to autoimmune disease?

Consider, for a moment, your digestive tract as a party: it's all the rage, lots of action, bacteria taking care of business, dancing the digestive boogie woogie…but it's exclusive, oh yes, selective, in fact.

Your intestinal membrane is like a big formidable bouncer, and if someone is not on the list, they don't get in.

Now imagine that your bouncer is tired of dealing with all the stress: damaging antibiotics are messing with the bacterial "cool kids," NSAIDS (Advil, aspirin, Tylenol, Alleve, etc.) are corroding the doors, and trigger happy toxins are looking for a fight.

Before you know it, he's stretched too thin, leaving the doors ajar and in walks all manner of riffraff. Now you've got a problem. Security hustles over in the form of your immune system, and in the chaos things start getting out of control. It's a domino effect of friendly fire, toxic overload, body out of whack.

That's leaky gut syndrome, a modern ailment and a physiological indicator of the toxic world our bodies have to deal with.

Leaky gut is a malady that is not widely accepted as an official medical condition, yet a growing body of research supports the concern that practitioners of whole-body health care have been voicing for years.

Through studies and investigations it is becoming clear that when your intestinal lining becomes too permeable, the effects of the unwanted toxins and particles in your intestines have a ripple effect across your entire body.

Leaky gut is also now thought to be linked to autoimmune disease because it causes your immune system to go into overdrive. And once your body crosses over into full blown disease, there is often no turning back.

How Does Leaky Gut Happen?

When the lining of the digestive tract is inflamed, the connections between the pieces of lining known as "tight junctions" break down and allow large, undigested compounds—toxins and bacteria—to leak into the bloodstream.

These substances all react with the intestine's immune system and cause an exaggerated immune response. This over-reaction by the immune system becomes a vicious cycle that leads to more intestinal damage.

And as this problem grows, diet, lifestyle, medications, and infections can cause further intestinal inflammation that can ultimately lead to more serious problems.

In addition, after the intestinal lining becomes damaged, the damaged cells become unable to properly digest food and produce the enzymes necessary for digestion.

This damage can lead to malnutrition, further intestinal inflammation, further permeability challenges, the development of food sensitivities, bacteria and yeast overgrowths, and an impaired immune system leading to irritable bowel syndrome, Crohn's disease, and other auto-immune diseases like Hashimoto's.

These self-destructive patterns can be very difficult to unwind.

> ## *Leaky gut is something that must be addressed*

Why Does This Matter?

I hope that by now you have a sense of how all of these different systems are connected and that this is way more than a thyroid problem.

Well, leaky gut, in my opinion, is a kind of fulcrum or nexus of all these systems and this is where autoimmune disease begins, where it progresses and the place that can make the most difference in your healing process.

Here's the thing, it also is not static. It is constantly progressing and many of the problems in other systems of your body are connected to the gut and like any fulcrum, this is a place of maximum leverage.

Things can quickly go from bad to worse. And they can go much more quickly in the direction of healing if you focus on fixing all the factors that lead to leaky gut.

But this requires a steadfast commitment to fostering good health in the gut. In essence, you must become a farmer of your gut ecosystem. Just like a farmer must plant, seed, fertilize and cultivate his crops and his farm, you need to do this for your gut.

In the beginning of the book, I shared about the 80/20 principle. Well, in my opinion, leaky gut and what is happening in the ecosystem of your gut are the top 5-10 percent.

This is arguably the most important area and if you get nothing else from this book I want you to come away with an understanding of this. The factors that lead to leaky gut contain the seeds of healing (and remission) in them.

So, of course this begs the question: What are these factors?

Diet, insulin resistance (sugar addiction), low stomach acid, adrenal stress, (which can lead directly to hypothyroidism), imbalance of healthy bacteria, poor fat digestion, constipation, problems with estrogen building up in the body.

So, what needs to be done to fix this?

Firstly, the diet. I explore the Autoimmune Paleo diet below. This diet works for leaky gut because it removes many of the offending foods that drive further destruction of the gut.

Gluten dairy, soy, seeds, nuts, beans, other grains, nightshades (and add common medications like antacids and NSAIDS). Some people see this and just want to give up or they start negotiating how they can get around eliminating some of these things.

Well, think about it this way. If I told you that you could make a single investment and double, triple or even 10x your money if you stuck with it. Wouldn't you want to make that investment? And if you did double, triple or 10x your money wouldn't you put more money into it?

That's what this diet is. It's a way getting a great return on your investment. Now, it's not magic and there are other factors that can get in the way and make it less effective and make the investment not work as well for you.

Factors That Undermine Success

Insulin resistance: We've already covered sugar issues. This is a key issue and often people with Hashimoto's use sugar to overcome fatigue. They also use sugar or carbohydrates as comfort food to try and overcome the emotional pain, anxiety and depression.

I know because I've done this and still struggle with it, at times. But this can lead to adrenal stress because the adrenals release cortisol to try and compensate for excess sugar and, ultimately it undermines gut health.

Low stomach acid: We've already touched on this, as well.. This affects everything downstream. And one of the consequences of this is further destruction of the gut.

172

Adrenal stress: We'll explore this in depth in the chapters on the Water Element. High cortisol leads to further destruction of the immune barrier, can degenerate the intestinal walls, and can promote more inflammation in the gut. (Interesting side note: steroid therapy used for inflammation can also do the same things).

Imbalance of healthy bacteria: This is a huge issue in the way that it influences the thyroid and Hashimoto's. The toxins released by bacteria can reduce thyroid hormone levels, contribute to thyroid hormone receptor resistance, decrease TSH, increase the amount of inactive T3, and make Hashimoto's worse.

Problems with fat digestion: We'll take a more in depth look at the gall bladder when in the chapters on the Wood Element, but I just want to mention it here as well. When fat isn't broken down and digested properly it can lead to further inflammation and breakdown in the gut because these fats can become rancid.

In addition, good fat is important as a building block for steroid hormones like estrogen, progesterone, testosterone and cortisol. It also transports important minerals and is essential for the absorption and storage of key vitamins like Vitamins A, D, E and K.

Slow transit through the gut: One factor that's a very common problem with people with Hashimoto's is that everything slows down in the gut. This can result in constipation, more inflammation and more problems with gut bacteria.

In the ecosystem of the gut everything is, of course, also connected. And things slowly down can lead to fermentation, fats going rancid and bacteria getting out of control and out of balance.

Too much estrogen: Another issue that you may think about being related to the gut and Hashimoto's is how it can contribute to excess estrogen in the body. A clogged liver due to excess sugar and gall bladder issues and problems caused by poor digestion and bacterial overgrowth can all lead to the buildup of excess estrogen to the point where it can actually become toxic.

This creates another vicious cycle because excess estrogen can cause an increase in thyroid binding globulin and this means less thyroid hormone can be freed to get into the cells and we wind up with another contributor to "functional hypothyroidism".

173

What Happens When the Intestines Break Down?

As we have already discussed, leaky gut leads to body-wide inflammation and pain. The tissues that get inflamed vary with different people and seem to depend on genetics and environmental factors.

This cycle of suffering can lead to:

- Gluten sensitivity and Celiac disease

- Food allergies

- Inflammatory bowel diseases

- Autoimmune diseases

- Neurological conditions

- Cognitive problems (depression, anxiety, Schizophrenia) and more

That last bullet is critical, recent research has revealed the remarkably strong connection between the brain and the intestines. In fact, the brain and gut are highly integrated and they communicate with each other, mostly through the autonomic nervous system (ANS) and the hypothalamus pituitary adrenal (HPA) axis.

It is also interesting to note that main area that controls the gut in the brain is the limbic system which is very much connected to our emotions and feelings. The nervous system of the gut is so sophisticated it is sometimes referred to as a second brain.

And permeability and inflammation in the intestines has been shown to directly lead to permeability and inflammation in the brain, as well. "As above, so below" is certainly true of the brain and the intestines.

What Is the Best Test for Leaky Gut?

Twenty years ago, many people measured leaky gut by measuring leakage of a sugar molecule (lactalose) into the blood stream. Since then, researchers and doctors in clinical practice have questioned this practice because very small molecules like sugar do not really challenge the immune system effectively.

174

They decided that we needed a better way to look at the breakdown of the barrier system.

Cyrex labs developed a test that does several things: it looks at what triggers the breakdown of the intestines, such as toxins produced by bacteria and antibodies produced against parts of the intestine's barrier system, such as occludin, zonulin, and actomysin.

Here are the four things that we test for intestinal permeability and why they matter. I touched on this test in Chapter 2. Cyrex Labs calls it **Array # 2—** the test for leaky gut.

Various proteins give us valuable information on how the gut is breaking down

1. Lipopolysaccharides (LPS): These are large molecules found in certain bacteria. They are toxins produced by gram-negative bacteria and, if they are absorbed, they cause a strong immune response. If antibodies against LPS are found, this shows that large molecules have leaked through the intestinal barrier into the bloodstream.

2. Occludin: This is a protein that holds together the tight junctions of the intestines. It's like glue that binds cells together. If antibodies to occludin are found, it shows that these junctions are breaking down. This is a way to measure the breakdown of the intestinal barrier membrane.

3. Zonulin: This is a protein that regulates how easily things can pass through the walls of the intestines. It's like a zipper. If antibodies to zonulin are found, it shows that the normal process that regulates the passage of all kinds of stuff through the intestines is compromised. The zipper has opened up the cells. This can be a clue to what may be causing the damage to the barrier system.

Zonulin has recently become popular in drug manufacturing and a new generation of drugs will have this protein added to insure that the medication is more easily absorbed. It's a bit frightening when you think about the implications.

4. The Actomysin Network: This is a group of proteins that controls the intestine's barrier system by maintaining the flexibility of the tight junctions. This is kind of like the anchor of the intestines. If antibodies to the actomysin network are found, it shows there is a problem with the barrier system by infiltrating cells.

For example, 92 percent of celiac disease patients with flat intestinal mucosa have antibodies to actin. This test measures the mechanism involved in damaging the intestinal barrier.

Ok, that's a lot of information on leaky gut.

Let's shift gears and take a look at some solution.

The Autoimmune Diet:
An Excellent Foundation for Healing

Much has been written about the Autoimmune Paleo Diet. It is a simplified approach that removes many of the most inflammatory foods from your diet.

In the beginning there is an elimination phase which cuts out gluten, dairy, soy, eggs, nuts, seeds, beans, all grains and nightshades.

This is truly healing though subtraction and it helps reduces systemic inflammation by eliminating (for a period of time) all the foods that may irritate and further exacerbate irritation and destruction of the intestinal lining.

Much of the difficulty that people have in healing Hashimoto's comes from its complexity. And simplifying and removing variables can be quite helpful in getting to the root of the problem.

This is difficult for many people to understand and is antithetical to a consumer culture where pills, supplements and other quick solutions are being marketed and sold by the millions daily.

But, despite its simplicity and the challenge of cutting out all these foods, it is remarkably effective in calming the immune system and providing the body with an opportunity to heal.

I advocate the Elimination Diet from the Autoimmune Paleo protocol as an excellent first step in calming immune function and beginning the process of healing the gut. This diet comes from my teacher, Dr. Datis Kharrazian, and from others like, Dr. Sarah Ballantyne, known as Paleo Mom.

Those of you who have worked with me know that I am also a big fan of Mickey Trescott, and we've been using her book as a starting point. In her book, *The Autoimmune Paleo Cookbook*, is an excellent list of foods to include and foods to avoid.

The entire purpose of this approach is to get things back in balance. It is also an excellent time to use targeted nutrition to support the liver in detoxification, to heal the intestinal lining and to restore the ecosystem of the gut. In addition, it can be quite helpful as foundation for reducing inflammation and neurodegeneration in the brain.

The Autoimmune Paleo Diet

• **Eliminates a lot of foods that cause problems in the digestive tract**

• **Helps reset your body from the whole sugar burner/sugar addict mode to a fat burning mode**

• **Gives you a chance to repair and rebuild your digestive tract as you do it**

• **And it can dramatically improve the results of the supplements and medication you are taking because it also improves absorption and utilization of these nutrients.**

It really is the foundation for success.

People become so used to certain foods that they sometimes don't realize those foods are harming them.

Instead, they believe a foggy brain, skin rashes or rosacea, chronic respiratory issues, joint pain, water retention, a distended belly, chronic digestive issues, and lots of other symptoms are a normal part of life.

Foods that most commonly trigger these reactions are gluten, dairy, eggs, corn, soy, and yeast. Sometimes nuts are also a problem. And, technically, a person can develop an intolerance to any food, especially one that is eaten repeatedly when leaky gut is an issue.

So it is recommended to eliminate all these foods and do a few more things; like some repairing and rebuilding. After that you can reintroduce foods slowly and systematically to identify which foods are triggers that lead to immune reactions. It is recommend to reintroduce one food for three days and keep track of what happens.

It's Important to Keep Track

This is why I asked you to keep a journal. You need to observe your reactions: these can be physical, psychological, and emotional. We've seen how emotions are so interconnected with these organ systems.

Another thing that's important to note is that adverse reactions aren't a bad thing. Everything is just a test and whether something "works" and makes you feel better or "doesn't work" and makes you feel worse, that data is valuable because it is diagnostic.

This is the key component of the **Reassess and Readjust** part of the **A.P.A.R.T System.** You have to evaluate what you're doing and keep track of what works and what doesn't.

For example, if you react to a food, then you know that food can't be part of your diet. It may be that you still need to do more work, or it might simply mean you just can't handle it.

You can revisit that food in a few more months, but you have to be prepared to say good-bye to some of these foods forever. Gluten, of course, is one of them.

Also, as we've established, digestive health is very much linked to blood sugar balance.

The other benefit to this elimination diet is that it is low carb in nature. This has the double benefit of repairing leaky gut and of balancing blood sugar.

If you have any of the following key symptoms, you may need to get this carbohydrate issue under control: insomnia, or waking up at 3:00 am or 4:00 am, an energy crash in the late afternoon, feeling spacey, irritable, or light headed if you go too long without eating, constant hunger, constant craving for sweets, and difficulty losing weight.

Sugar imbalance also leads to many hormonal problems, not just the thyroid. It impacts the adrenals, estrogen and progesterone levels, and more. If you have any of the symptoms mentioned above, you may have hypoglycemia, insulin resistance, or some combination of both.

And that's a lot to obsess about! (Remember over-thinking is a symptom of an out of balanced Earth Element.)

Other Infections that Can Also Cause Problems

To wind things up, let's take a look at a couple of other factors that we haven't really gotten into yet regarding digestive health.

These infections of the digestive tract can greatly complicate this whole process, and they're something that you need to look at and evaluate.

1. Parasites: These little critters are quite common. Some of the ones we have seen are amoeba, Giardia, roundworms, and pinworms.

They can cause problems such as bowel irregularities like diarrhea, constipation or IBS like symptoms, anemia, skin conditions, insomnia, emotional issues, immune dysfunction and they can prevent other healing processes.

A stool test is the best laboratory test to determine whether or not you have parasites.

Herbs can sometimes be effective in treating parasitic infections. However, with a really tenacious parasite, you may need to use medication. It can sometimes be quicker, more effective, and easier on you in the long run.

Clinical Pearl: As with any medical decision you must always do a risk-benefit analysis. What's the risk of using a particular drug, herb, supplement, therapy or surgery? Then you need to ask what the benefit is.

The benefit should always outweigh the risk and the best decisions are usually those in which the benefit outweighs the risk by a wide margin.

2. Yeast overgrowth—Candida: Candida is a rather popular diagnosis among many practitioners and has been linked to a number of health problems.

But, in my opinion, you have to be cautious when treating Candida. Some of the anti-fungal treatments that are recommended are very hard on the liver and can wipe out some of the good flora in the gut.

This is a good example of the benefit not always being as good as advertized. And the risk is that you destroy some important good bacteria in the process.

So, my suggestion is to test for Candida and act accordingly. Antibiotic overuse can lead to Candida overgrowth and so can the high carb, high sugar diet that we've been talking about in this chapter.

And instead of the harsh Candida attack, one of the best approaches to healing this condition is the diet that we have just discussed, the Elimination diet with added emphasis on eliminating sugars.

That's a simple approach where the benefit clearly outweighs the risk.

Don't you just love elegant solutions? I do. Whenever, as a practitioner, I can find something that does multiple good things at once, I rejoice.

So let's take a moment to rejoice! Yeah, elegant solutions!

3. Bacterial overgrowth of species that are not helping us, such as H. Pylori.

A few different kinds of bacterial overgrowth are located in different places. In the stomach is Heliobactor Pylori, or H. Pylori. This bacteria is linked to gastritis, heartburn, and nausea. Over 80 percent of the people who have it are asymptomatic.

Some believe it actually has a purpose and is beneficial if it doesn't get out of control. Herbs are really effective in treating this, particularly those containing berberine.

In the small intestine, we have SIBO, or Small Intestinal Bacterial Overgrowth. The chapter on the Fire element will explain more about SIBO.

In an earlier chapter on the large intestine, we discussed the acronym FODMAP, which sounds a bit like a bad corporation. "Yes, I'm the senior

180

VP over at FODMAP. We produce natural gas."

Not Bacteria, Exactly, But Related

As you may recall,. FODMAP foods are poorly digested in the small intestine, and bacteria love to ferment them so that they can have their own party!

This fermentation results in gas in the large intestines and other complaints. I've included a whole article on it in the supplemental section on our website.. A lot of the problem foods in that list are also eliminated with the Elimination diet. So this brings cause for more celebration.

So, all of this begs the question: How do we figure out this intestinal condition? And what do we do about it?

The best way to test for all of these issues is to do a comprehensive stool test. A number of labs offer these and they test for all the critters that we mentioned above, and some test for some gluten antibodies as well.

As the name implies, it's quite comprehensive and will give us a lot of helpful data about the state of the ecosystem that lives in your gut.

Then what do we do?

We do a four-step protocol I call "**Farming Your Gut**":

Being a Good Gut Farmer

Here is a strategy for maintaining the gut's ecosystem like a good farmer watches over his or her farm. (**Weed, Compost, Plant, & Heal**) For a more detailed description of this strategy see the supplemental section of our website: https://hashimotos-diet.com/roadmap-to-remission-supplemental/

The four steps are:

1. Weed: Remove the bad guys we mentioned above: the parasites, fungi/yeast and bad bacterial species using herbs and supplements or medication, if necessary.

2. Compost: Replace important stuff like enzymes, bile and HCL, etc.

in the ecosystem.

3. Plant: Repopulate the good guys; like more good bacteria.

4. Heal the terrain: Repair the ecosystem and the intestinal lining.

I advocate healing while weeding, especially if you have identified that you have leaky gut.

Important Takeways

1. The Earth element is the spleen/pancreas and stomach, and to some degree, the entire digestive tract.

2. The negative emotion of the Earth element is obsessive thinking or worry. The positive attributes are integrity and giving back in a healthy way.

3. Blood sugar balance is hugely important for healing Hashimoto's. Ignore this at your peril. I don't want to play with you if you won't fix this.

4. Leaky gut, and other intestinal issues like parasites, Candida yeast, and bacterial overgrowth also need to be evaluated and dealt with.

5. The Elimination phase of the Autoimmune Paleo diet is an elegant solution in that it addresses so many of the issues we talked about today and it is a great foundation for the other things we are doing. It's not the total answer, but it increases your chances of success dramatically.

6. There is no such thing as "sort of gluten-free". It's just like being an alcoholic. You can't be "sort of sober."

Chapter Twelve

Using the A.P.A.R.T. System to Heal the Earth Element

The A.P.A.R.T. System

Applying the A.P.A.R.T. System to the Earth Element

Alright, great stuff. Now let's apply the **A.P.A.R.T.** System to the Earth element.

Take out your journal and look for symptoms of problems with the Earth Element. Note what they are, then create a plan for addressing them. After that, you must act on your plan. Follow through and do what you have planned.

After that take inventory of what you did. Look at what worked and what didn't. Both will provide valuable information.

Double down on what worked, change what didn't. Keep doing it.

Since the Earth Element is a kind of fulcrum, this should be an ongoing process that you do all year round.

1. A = Ask and Assess: *Signs and Symptoms*

Stomach: (Both sets of symptoms could be caused by too little stomach acid.)

Too Little Stomach Acid

Excessive belching, burping, or bloating; gas immediately following a meal; offensive breath, difficult bowel movements, sense of fullness during and after meals, difficulty digesting fruits and vegetables; and undigested food found in stools.

Feeling of Too Much Stomach Acid (Often Caused by Too Little)

These symptoms may, at their root, be caused by too little stomach acid. So boosting stomach acid is still an important part of the solution. But you may need to do some healing first. The Autoimmune approach can be quite helpful here as well.

Stomach pain, burning, or aching one to four hours after eating; feel hungry an hour or two after eating; Heartburn when lying down or bending forward; temporary relief by using antacids, food, milk, or carbonated beverages; digestive problems subside with rest and relaxation; heartburn due to spicy foods, chocolate, citrus, peppers, alcohol, and caffeine.

Blood Sugar Issues

Hypoglycemia:

Crave sweets during the day; irritable if meals are missed; depend on coffee to keep going/get started; get light-headed if meals are missed; eating relieves fatigue; feel shaky, jittery, or have tremors; agitated, easily upset, or nervous; poor memory/forgetful; blurred vision.

186

Insulin Resistance:

Fatigue after meals; crave sweets during the day; eating sweets does not relieve cravings for sugar; must have sweets after meals; waist girth is equal or larger than hip girth; frequent urination, increased thirst and appetite; difficulty losing weight.

Leaky Gut Symptoms:

Leaky gut is often the foundation of much larger systemic problems and diseases. It can lead to:

1. Digestive problems like gas, bloating, diarrhea and IBS like symptoms.

2. Allergic reactions or hyper allergic responses

3. Autoimmune diseases – in fact, I would go far as to say that leaky gut is ground zero for autoimmune disease. It is an essential ingredient for the formation and progression of these diseases.

4. Chronic Fatigue and Fibromyalgia

5. Mood disorders and cognitive problems like anxiety, depression, ADD and ADHD. Because there is such a strong connection between the brain and the gut, many neurological disorders are also caused by leaky gut.

6. Skin problems, rashes, dermatitis, acne and more.

Order a Comprehensive Stool Test

Those are all the symptoms, as we discussed previously a comprehensive stool test can also give you information on parasites, yeast/fungi, problem bacterial species, leaky gut, malabsorption and more.

2. P = Prioritize and Plan

Not everything has the same level of importance. This is what 80/20 teaches us. Some things are having more of an impact than others. Figure out which they are (the positive feedback loops) and then make a plan to fix them.

So you must decide, which of the Earth systems have been compromised? The stomach, the spleen/pancreas, the gut?

Here's the thing; it could be all of them. If it is, heal all of them.

187

3. A = Act and Adapt

Act and put your plan into motion, then observe what the results are. Double down on what works and change what doesn't. Results should be apparent relatively quickly. If they aren't, you need to make changes.

Blood Sugar Regulation

How to Keep Blood Sugar in A Healthy Range

When balancing blood sugar, there are two things to think about. The first is fasting blood glucose, which you can measure first thing in the morning before eating or drinking anything.

In functional medicine we define normal range for fasting blood glucose as somewhere between 75 – 95 mg/dL. (Although 100 is often considered the top of the range for normal, studies have shown that fasting blood sugar levels at the high end of normal may set you up for diabetes in the future.) This is another one of those instances where numbers are numbers and there are various factors that can impact what the numbers mean.

And although 80 mg/dL is often defined as low end of the range, there are healthy people with a fasting blood sugar in the mid-to-high 70s (especially if they follow a low-carb diet—all you Paleo fans—time to do the wave).

The second, and more important thing to measure your blood sugar one to two hours after a meal. This is called "post-prandial" blood glucose.

Studies have shown that post-prandial blood glucose may be a more accurate predictor of future diabetes (as well as cardiovascular disease) and may also be a better initial marker -before blood tests like fasting blood glucose and Hemoglobin A 1 C (Hb1Ac) to indicate blood sugar imbalances.

Normal blood sugar one to two hours after a meal is 120 mg/dL, but most normal people are under 100 mg/dL two hours after a meal.

How This Applies to You

How does this apply to you? If you're hypoglycemic, your challenge is to keep your blood sugar above 75 throughout the day.

The best way to do this is to eat a low-to-moderate carbohydrate diet –the Autoimmune Paleo diet is ideal for this(to prevent the blood sugar spikes and crashes I discussed above), and to eat frequent, small meals every two to three hours (to ensure a continuous supply of energy to the body).

If you're insulin resistant, your challenge is to keep your blood sugar below 120 two hours after a meal.

The only way you're going to be able to do this is to restrict carbohydrates.

Buy a Blood Glucose Meter

Everyone should buy a blood glucose meter. The technology has gotten to the point where they are very precise and quite inexpensive.

How low-carb do you need to go?

It's different for everyone. (But, for most people with Hashimoto's, it is recommended to reduce carbs significantly. However, as with most things there are exceptions to this rule and some people may find that they need a certain amount of carbohydrates to function properly.

If this is the case it is recommended to incorporate resistant starches, which are starches that release sugar more slowly and don't give you a dramatic spike in blood sugar.)

First, figure out your carbohydrate tolerance by buying a blood glucose meter and testing your blood sugar after various meals.

If you've eaten too many carbs, your blood sugar will remain above 120 mg/dL two hours after your meal.

Again, if you have Hashimoto's, it's also important that you take steps to make sure your thyroid is properly balanced as well.

As you have seen, this thing works in both directions.

Sugar problems can mess with thyroid function, and thyroid disorders like Hashimoto's can cause sugar problems and put you at greater risk for hypoglycemia, insulin resistance, and if nothing is corrected, diabetes.

So take blood sugar balance seriously. I mean it.

189

Some Foods that benefit the Earth Element

Earth: Spleen/Pancreas

Food Suggestions:

Deficient spleen-pancreas qi—congee (soup made from rice), oats, sweet rice, pounded sweet rice. Carb rich vegetables—winter squash, carrot, rutabaga, parsnip, turnip, garbanzo beans, black beans, peas, sweet potato, yam, pumpkin._Pungent vegetables and spices—onion, leek, black pepper, ginger, cinnamon, fennel, garlic, nutmeg, small amounts of certain sweeteners and cooked fruits—rice syrup, molasses, cherry, and date.

For severe deficiency—small amounts of animal foods prepared in soup or congee—mackerel, tuna, halibut, anchovy, beef, beef liver or kidney, chicken, turkey, or lamb.

Foods that dry dampness (overproduction of mucus)—aduki beans, celery, lettuce, pumpkin, scallion, alfalfa, turnip, kohlrabi, white pepper, raw honey.

> *Clinical Pearl:*
> *Soup and broth, like bone broth, are some of the most healing foods for the Earth element. If you want to heal your gut, eat more soup.*

Blood Sugar Regulation

Foods Commonly used in the Treatment of Diabetes

- Grains and Legumes (Not recommended in the Elimination Phase of the Autoimmune Diet)—millet, rice, sweet rice, oats, fresh corn, , mung bean, garbanzo bean

- Chlorophyll Foods—spirulina, chlorella, liquid chlorphyll

- Vegetables and fruits—string bean, carrot, radish, Jerusalem artichoke, turnip, asparagus, yam, spinach, avocado, pear, plum, lemon, grapefruit, lime, blueberry, huckleberry

- Herbs—dandelion root and leaf, cedar berries, yarrow flowers, blueberry/huckleberry leaf

- Sweeteners—licorice tea or powder

- Animal Products—Clams, albalone, lamb pancreas, pork, beef or fowl, lamb kidney, chicken or goose, beef

Qi Gong for the Earth Element:
Between Heaven and Earth

Between Heaven and Earth

This exercise balances and harmonizes and heals the entire digestive system. The movement of the hands in opposite directions pulls and lifts the stomach, spleen, liver and gall bladder.It is an effective exercise for constipation because it stimulates peristalsis and helps to bring blood flow to the intestines, as well.

Begin in the natural standing form, feet shoulder width apart, hands hanging relaxed at your side. Bring your hands up to your belly, just below your navel gathering a ball of energy.

Inhale, and continue to bring your hands up to your solar plexus (just below your heart). As you exhale, separate your palms.

Rotate your right palm up and towards the sky and your left palm down and towards the ground. Rise up on your tip toes if your balance allows. Your eyes and your head should follow your right hand upwards.

Move the plams in these opposite directions until the right arm is fully extended above the head. Point your fingers towards the left and bend your palm at a 90 degree angle as though you were holding a small stone in your hand.

The left hand should also be at a 90 degree angle and should be extended downward towards the earth and point forward. Try to get your hands to 90 degrees, but if you aren't flexible enough just go as far as you can comfortably.

In your mind visualize your opposite hands connecting energetically to heaven and to earth. In Chinese medicine man (or woman) is considered to exist in the pace between heaven and earth.

Inhale as you return your arms towards your body, facing both palms downward towards the ground.

Exhale and gently push both hands down, visualize negative energy flowing out of you and down into the earth.

Finish by returning your hands to the starting position just below your navel. One palm on top of the other.

Repeat the entire exercise on the opposite side.

*Repeat 3 times on each side one to three times a day.

Want to see a video demonstration of this form? Visit our supplemental page at https://hashimotos-diet.com/roadmap-to-remission-supplemental/

4. R= Reassess and Readjust

Retest, reassess, and ask all over again. Figure out what worked and what didn't. Double down on what worked and either eliminate or recreate a plan for what didn't.

With the Earth Element journaling is an absolute necessity. Once you remove foods for a period of time and then reintroduce them you'll want to keep track of this process.

It is best to reintroduce 1 food at a time, so that is your only variable and to test it for 3 consecutive days. Note anything and everything in your journal. You will know if it is a food that you can't reintroduce because you will feel absolutely terrible after eating it.

5. T = Try and Try Again

Keep doing it, keep refining, keep building on the positive results and keep looking for the remaining positive feedback loops that are causing vicious cycles.

Build on all your victories. Celebrate them and use them to create more positive momentum.

Chapter Thirteen

The Water Element:
The Root of Healing

In this chapter you will learn about the water element—another system that is incredibly important for healing. The water element includes the kidneys, the adrenals, and the urinary bladder.

The kidneys and the adrenals play a huge role in unravelling the Hashimoto's puzzle.

With the Water element an entirely different set of vicious cycles are at work, and a systematical approach will help to unwind them.

And, by now, you should be starting to get a real sense of what we're up against.

Hashimoto's is a formidable foe. You aren't going to fix it with some cookie-cutter approach or one supplement or one drug. It's too involved, it's too complicated, and it's not always linear.

The vicious cycles that we have seen so far all feed on one another, so there are times when you have exponential decline, and if you start repairing and unwinding them and you stay vigilant and committed, you start to see exponential progress as well.

But, it doesn't end when you put down this book. First of all, what I have shared with you has taken years and years of research, study, and clinical experience.

You need to review this material, and keep learning. Visit our supplemental section and go deeper.

We have only begun to start unwinding these various systems and their vicious cycles. This takes committed work and, dare I say it, devotion.

Don't Be Discouraged, If I Can Do It So Can You

If you're feeling discouraged or overwhelmed, I totally get that, because I have been there. I have experienced many of these symptoms and challenges and I have been forced to walk the talk. So I understand the challenge.

You know, a few years ago I hit a major wall and I crashed. I was in pain all the time. I had no energy, I was depressed, and had such bad brain fog and memory issues that I really thought I was losing it.

I had to go through this process myself, do the evaluations, and change my diet. I follow the diet I introduced to you to this day. I journal, I take some supplements and I constantly have to be vigilant and committed. So I get it.

But I can also tell you this. The rewards are amazing. I feel so much better today. As long as I stay on track, I generally feel the best I have in 20 years or more..

And I want this for you too! But I also want you to know it takes some work. There are going to be challenges and setbacks.

You're going to need support and encouragement, don't try and do it all alone. Reach out and ask for help if you need it.

Allright, let's get into this chapter.

Here's what you'll learn:

- How thyroid health is intertwined with adrenal health. We'll explore the understanding of the endocrine system in Chinese medicine and how this impacts you emotionally and spiritually.

- We'll look at how the thyroid impacts kidney function.

- And, you'll learn how blood sugar balance is also critical for adrenal health and how these two systems are also interconnected.

Like I said in the last chapter, you can't escape the blood sugar reality. It is always going to be there and it has to be dealt with on a daily basis.

The Kidneys

The Water Element

In Chinese medicine the Water element is the kidneys and the urinary bladder. Both of these organs primarily function using liquids and water.So it's not a big leap to see how that connection was made.

Let's start with the kidneys. What do they do in the body? A lot.

Once again, when you really have a look, it's astonishing how our bodies work. The kidneys are considered, perhaps, the most important organ for homeostasis or natural balance in the body.

They are a two of the body's elimination channels as well as two of its regulatory organs. If the kidneys can not remove waste, toxins stay in the body and the body is forced to try and eliminate them through other channels.

One example of this would be the skin. The skin is also an organ of elimination, excreting uric acid and waste products in sweat and oil.

If the kidneys are not functioning at full strength, toxins will be eliminated through the skin. This may result in rashes, as irritating toxins are excreted through the skin. This may also result in strong urine like body odor.

Kidneys Regulate Chemical Balance

The kidneys also regulate chemical balance and water content in the body. If the kidneys are not performing that job, numerous health problems and symptoms can arise.

Some examples of these types of conditions are: gout (formation of uric acid crystals in the joints and kidneys), acidosis (a systemic problem of too much acid throughout the body), kidney and urinary bladder infections, and kidney stones.

The kidneys also provide an important function in maintaining fluid and electrolyte balance. Electrolytes are substances, such as salts, that dissolve or break down into ions when mixed with water. Optimal health depends on maintaining proper water and electrolyte balance.

Our bodies are 75 percent water. Water is used by every cell in the body and is essential for proper metabolism, because it provides the medium in which virtually all chemical reactions take place.

If the body has too much water, the kidneys excrete it. If we have too little, the kidneys conserve it by retaining it. It really is the organ of the Water element.

It is interesting to note that dehydration can cause you to experience pain in your kidneys. Some people incorrectly think that they have a lower back problem because of muscle stiffness or spinal problems when, in reality, they just need to drink more water.

Water Benefits the Water Element: Go Figure!

So next time your back hurts, try drinking water before you reach for that ibuprofen or acetaminophen (both of which can damage the kidneys, liver, and your intestines.)

The kidneys also keep the electrolytes in the body fluids in a sensitive balance. They regulate the levels of many chemical substances in the blood such as chloride, sodium, potassium, and bicarbonate.

The kidneys also regulate the balance between water and salt by selectively

198

keeping or excreting both substances as the body demands.

The kidneys maintain the blood's acid-alkaline balance, as do the lungs. Normal blood pH is between 7.45 and 7.35, and this is slightly alkaline. If the blood becomes too acidic or too alkaline, serious health consequences and even death may result.

The kidneys maintain this balance by controlling the absorption and replacement of certain ions (i.e., bicarbonate). Our diet and lifestyle choices can influence our body's acidity.

The Kidneys Regulate Blood Pressure

The kidneys also function in blood pressure regulation. When blood pressure is low, cells in the kidneys release a hormone that initiates a process that results in the constriction of blood vessels. This is part of the renin-angiotensin system.

The renin-angiotensin system (RAS) is a hormone system that regulates blood pressure and water (fluid) balance. When blood volume is low, the kidneys secrete renin. Renin stimulates the production of angiotensin.

Angiotensin causes blood vessels to constrict resulting in increased blood pressure. Erythropoietin is also produced in the kidneys, and when it passes through the bone marrow, erythropoietin binds to certain cells, stimulating them to create red blood cells.

The Kidneys Activate Vitamin D

Vitamin D is a group of fat-soluble hormones.

Its major role is to increase the flow of calcium into the bloodstream by promoting absorption of calcium and phosphorus from food in the intestines, and re-absorption of calcium in the kidneys, enabling normal mineralization of bone and preventing conditions caused by too little calcium. It is also necessary for bone growth and bone remodeling.

So why is Vitamin D so important for Hashimoto's?

It is important because Vitamin D deficiency has been linked to numerous autoimmune diseases such as rheumatoid arthritis, lupus, diabetes, multiple sclerosis and more in research studies.

Vitamin D plays an important role in balancing the TH-1 (cell-mediated) and

TH-2 humoral) arms of the immune system. It does this by influencing T-regulatory (TH-3) cells, which govern the expression and differentiation of TH-1 and TH-2 cells.

Remember in the chapter on the Metal Element, TH-3 is like the general of the immune system, calling back and calming down the troops. We need it to strengthen the command and control structure of the immune system.

Vitamin D deficiency is also specifically associated with autoimmune thyroid disease (AITD), and has been shown to benefit autoimmune mediated thyroid problems.

Vitamin D also has another lesser-known role. It regulates insulin secretion and sensitivity, and it balances blood sugar. As previously explained, insulin resistance and blood sugar problems mess with the thyroid in a number of ways.

Things that Reduce Vitamin D

Research over the last 20 years has identified a number of things that reduce the absorption, production, and activity of Vitamin D in the body. These include: latitude, air pollution, use of sunscreen, skin color, age, weight, skin temperature, and the health of your kidneys, liver and your gut.

Since Vitamin D is absorbed in the small intestine, guess what impacts its absorption? Yes, it's true, leaky gut can slow absorption of vitamin D.

High cortisol levels, which we will cover in a few minutes (caused by stress or medications like steroids), are also linked with lower vitamin D levels. The synthesis of active Vitamin D from sunlight depends on cholesterol.

Stress hormones are also made from cholesterol. When the body is in an active stress response, most of the cholesterol is used to make cortisol, and not enough cholesterol is left over for Vitamin D production.

Obesity reduces the activity of Vitamin D. Obese people have lower serum levels of it because it gets taken up by fat cells.

Not eating enough fat or not digesting fat properly reduces absorption of vitamin D. Vitamin D is a fat-soluble vitamin, which means it requires fat to be absorbed.

People on low-fat diets, and people with conditions that impair fat absorption (like IBS, IBD, gall bladder, or liver disease) are more likely to have low levels of Vitamin D.

A variety of drugs reduce absorption or biologic activity of Vitamin D. Unfortunately, these include drugs that are among the most popular and frequently prescribed—including antacids, replacement hormones, corticosteroids, anticoagulants, and blood thinners.

Aging reduces the conversion of sunlight to Vitamin D.

Inflammation of any type reduces the utilization of Vitamin D. And as we have learned, inflammation is at the root of our problems.

But Wait, There's More

To further complicate matters, we now know that certain people with normal levels of Vitamin D still suffer from deficiency symptoms.

How is this possible?

For circulating Vitamin D to perform its functions, it must first activate the Vitamin D receptor (VDR). The problem is that many people with autoimmune disease have a genetic defect that affects the expression and activation of the Vitamin D receptors and reduces the biologic activity of Vitamin D.

Studies have shown that a significant number of patients with autoimmune Hashimoto's disease have VDR defects. And we've seen this clinically many times, as well.

Here's what this means: if you have low thyroid function, you might be experiencing Vitamin D deficiency even if your blood levels of Vitamin D are normal.

It also means that, if you have a VDR polymorphism, it's likely you'll need to have higher than normal blood levels of vitamin D to avoid the effects of Vitamin D deficiency.

It's also important to be cautious here because too much Vitamin D can also be problematic. So this needs to be monitored. You need to assess and reassess.

As with many things in the body there is a "Goldilocks zone". Determining where your ideal zone is may take some trial and error, but a good general benchmark for 25 OH Vitamin D is between 55 to 70 NG/ml.

Yup, so much more than a thyroid problem, people.

Quick Recap

The kidneys do a whole lot:

- **They maintain fluid, electrolyte, and acid-alkaline balance.**

- **They eliminate metabolic wastes.**

- **They help regulate blood pressure.**

- **They produce a hormone that stimulates red blood cell production (erythropoietin or EPO)**

- **They activate Vitamin D**

Urinary Bladder

What about the urinary bladder? Its job is pretty straightforward.

The bladder is a hollow muscular organ shaped like a balloon. It sits in your pelvis and is held in place by ligaments attached to other organs and the pelvic bones.

The bladder stores urine until you are ready to go to the bathroom. It swells into a round shape when it is full and gets smaller when empty. If the urinary system is healthy, the bladder can hold up to 16 ounces (two cups) of urine comfortably for two to five hours.

The Hashimoto's Connection

Okay, what's the kidney and urinary bladder have to do with Hashimoto's?

You guessed it, Hashimoto's and hypothyroidism can have a big impact on both kidney and urinary bladder function.

> ### Hypothyroidism & Hashimoto's can cause:
>
> - **Less blood flow to the kidneys.** This can cause creatinine to build up and not be excreted. Creatinine is a chemical waste molecule that is generated from muscle metabolism.
>
> - **Increased amounts of uric acid.** Some 20–30 percent of gout patients have hypothyroidism. This is often linked with higher levels of creatinine.
>
> - **High blood pressure.** According to one study by Danzi et al, up to 40 percent of hypothyroid patients had high blood pressure.

Again, if the kidneys fail to filter waste products from your body properly when your pressure is low, then "angiotensin" is produced, which raises your blood pressure.

Also, a rise in cortisol from your adrenals can raise your blood pressure. Hypothyroidism can also cause edema. You can see this swelling under the eyes, or as mild swelling of the hands and feet. This is a very common symptom for people with Hashimoto's.

Swelling is caused by several things: decreased kidney function, capillaries becoming more permeable, poor lymphatic drainage, and salt and water retention by the kidneys.

Recap: Hypothyroidism and the Kidneys

Hypothyroidism can lead to alterations in salt and water, calcium, phosphate, Vitamin D and uric acid levels, high blood pressure, and edema.

It's all connected. Kidneys are the water organ.

The endocrine gland of the Water element is the adrenals. Now let's take a look at the adrenal glands.

Chapter Fourteen

The Adrenals

The adrenals are two little glands, about almond size, that sit on top of the kidneys. The one on the right kidney has a triangular shape and the one on the left kidney has a sort of half moon shape. (Perhaps this difference in shape of the 2 kidneys is what led ancient doctors to view give one kidney yin and the other yang attributes.)

Each of the adrenals has two different zones. The inner zone, or the medulla, secretes adrenalin and norepinephrine and just the right amount of dopamine. These are the stress hormones.

The outer zone…(imagine Rod Serling of The Twilight Zone doing the voice over for this next passage)

…You're traveling through another dimension—a dimension not only of sight and sound but of mind—a journey into a wondrous land whose boundaries are that of the imagination. That's a signpost up ahead: Your Next Stop…

… the outer zone—the adrenal cortex.

This is where three different types of hormones are secreted: glucocorticoids, mineralocorticoids, and androgens. These hormones are all made from cholesterol (See? It does do good things) and are critical to every day function.

Of the glucocorticoids, cortisol is the star. It is stimulated by ACTH from the pituitary. This is very much like the relationship between TSH (also secreted by the pituitary) and T4. ACTH and cortisol are the analogous hormones of the adrenals.

What does cortisol do? It regulates blood sugar levels, increases body fat, defends the body against infections, and helps the body adapt to stress. It also helps to convert food into energy and is anti-inflammatory.

What doesn't it do might be a better question. It's the body's fixer.

Aldosterone is the main mineralocorticoid. It helps regulate blood volume, blood pressure, and the body's sodium and potassium levels.

Androgen Hormones

The androgen hormones are testosterone and DHEA (which stands for the impossible to pronounce dehydroepiandrosterone).

These are present in both men and women. DHEA is popular for being the "youth hormone." It does have anti-aging effects. It also helps the body fight infections and helps protect the body from the effects of cortisol and stress.

Cholesterol gets converted into the precursor for all those hormones called pregnenolone. Pregnenolone is also a precursor for cortisol.

With chronic stress, the kind that causes a host of health problems, including hypothyroidism, something called a "pregnenolone steal" happens.

Here the body says, "Sorry, DHEA and testosterone, we need to borrow pregnenolone for a little while and use it to make more cortisol."

This is the body's way of conserving resources to help us survive stressful situations, like living with Hashimoto's. The problem with chronic stress is that we get stuck in a perpetual state of stress, and this ends up draining the adrenals.

Remember that because we're going to come back to it in a moment. I want to digress quickly into the brain. In Chapter 1, we talked a bit about the hypothalamus, where the ancient Taoists tapped into the energy of the big dipper.

The cosmos, the universe.

Hypothalamus: The boss of the boss

The hypothalamus is really like the boss of the boss. You know, like when the boss is real arrogant and always doing bossy things and then, all of a sudden, the boss's boss shows up and he gets put in his place?

Well the pituitary and the hypothalamus' relationship is nothing like that. (I just wanted to make sure you're paying attention.) Their relationship is more like, "Hey, we have this amazingly complex, super complicated body to run. Do you want to help each other? Cool!"

The hypothalamus is the pituitary's boss.

It says "Hey, pituitary, tell the liver to get his act together and while you're at it, tell the thyroid and the adrenals and the mammary glands and the ovaries. Tell them all the boss is back in town."

With the adrenals, this little benevolent enlightened dictatorship is called, the hypothalmic-pituitary-adrenal axis or the HPA axis. These three run the whole show.

The HPA axis plays a major role in regulating immune function, digestion, energy use, mood, and thrill of thrills, sexuality. This HPA axis is controlled by hormones (in a non-linear fashion) and it is totally manipulated by stress.

The Femme Fatale of the HPA Axis

Stress is like the femme fatale of the HPA axis. It's the mean wife of the boss' boss. You know, like the Leona Helmsley of the body. (She left 12 million dollars to her dog, named Trouble, when she died—12 million to a dog!)

Anyway, where am I going with all of this? A dysfunctional HPA axis, like a troubled empire ruled by the queen of mean, can cause all kinds of problems.

With Hashimoto's, one of the biggest reasons why people continue to feel exhausted even though they are taking thyroid hormones is because of a messed up HPA axis.

Here you may feel better initially and then you start feeling worse and worse, until you are right back to where you started, feeling like crap. And guess what?

The blood work looks normal or they have a low TSH and a low or low-normal T4.

Okay, so let's take a look at few different ways that stress, the Leona Helmsley of the body, causes hypothyroid symptoms:

Most people are aware of the obvious forms of stress that affect the adrenal glands: impossibly full schedules, driving in traffic, financial problems, divorce, losing a job, moving, and the many other emotional and psychological challenges of modern life.

But other things you don't normally think of also place just as much of a burden on the adrenal glands.

These include blood sugar swings, gut dysfunction, food intolerances (especially gluten), chronic infections, environmental toxins, autoimmune problems and inflammation.

All of these conditions sound the alarm bells and cause the adrenals to pump out more stress hormones. In this context, stress is broadly defined as "anything that disturbs the body's natural balance (homeostasis)."

Adrenal stress is probably the most common problem we encounter in clinical practice, because nearly everyone is dealing with at least one of the things I just discussed.

Symptoms of adrenal stress are many and nonspecific because the adrenals, like the thyroid, can affect every system in the body.

Common Symptoms of Adrenal Stress

Some of the more common symptoms are:

- Fatigue, also a thyroid symptom

- Eating to relieve fatigue, another blood sugar problem.

- Irritability or lightheadedness between meals—a blood sugar and adrenal problem.

- Mood swings

- Decreased immunity

- Dizziness when moving from sitting or lying to standing; it affects your blood pressure.

- Headaches, splitting headaches, especially

- Sleep issues. Difficulty falling asleep, staying asleep, and waking up feeling exhausted even after you had enough sleep.

- Sugar and caffeine cravings. Have a hankering for an iced frappacino? It could be your adrenals.

- Gastric ulcers. Ulcers in the stomach can be caused by the adrenals.

Weak adrenals can cause hypothyroid symptoms alone without any problem in the thyroid gland itself. In such cases, working on the adrenals themselves is the key to improving thyroid function.

The most significant indirect effect the adrenals have on thyroid function is via their influence on blood sugar.

High or low cortisol, caused by any of the chronic stressors listed above, can cause hypoglycemia, hyperglycemia, or both. And, as you learned in a previous chapter, blood sugar imbalances cause hypothyroid symptoms in a variety of ways.

But adrenal stress also has more direct impacts on thyroid function.

CASE STUDY: ADRENALS AS THE ROOT OF THE PROBLEM

A 29-year-old female who was diagnosed with Hashimoto's postpartum. (Used with permission)

She suffered from fatigue, brain fog, and concentration problems, muscle aches, and hip and shoulder pain. She also suffered mild depression and thinning hair and nails.

She had both Graves and Hashimoto's antibodies elevated, and high TSH (above 16 at one point). She fluctuated from hyper to hypo symptoms. She reported that these were "crazy cycles" for about 15 months.

She also could not tolerate thyroid replacement hormone at all. She had a very bad reaction to both Synthroid and Armour.

Further investigating revealed signs and symptoms of leaky gut, hypoglycemia, and adrenal issues, and high homocysteine levels.

We put her on an autoimmune diet, treated her hypoglycemia by making sure she started the day with a good protein and fat combination, and didn't let her sugar crash throughout the day. She ate at regular intervals.

We also treated the leaky gut and worked on the adrenals and helped her adapt to stressors. And we worked to aggressively reduce the systemic inflammation that's was at the root of this.

After working together for three months, she felt considerable improvement.

She returned to her primary physician, reported what she had done, and requested a follow-up blood test. This doctor initially refused because he said that it wasn't possible that there could be any improvement with that type of treatment.

Diet and the adrenals didn't matter, and so on. She insisted, and finally he relented and ordered the tests.

Everything came back within the normal range, (all the antibodies, the TSH, and everything else).

She was, of course, elated.

Here is an actual email she sent us:

"Hello Marc!

I know you didn't ask me for an update, but everyone deserves praise every now and then:)

Well this is... (her name),...and if you remember, you helped me about eighteen months ago. I had horrible antibodies, leaky gut, adrenal problems, etc. All of this came after a pregnancy.

Anyways, my thyroid antibodies have not come back, my gut feels amazing (unless I accidentally ingest gluten:)) and I assume my adrenals are working just fine! In fact, I'm pregnant again with my second, and my thyroid is looking good and I'm feeling amazing!!!

I owe this all to you!

So once again, thank you so much, you literally changed my life, and keep the Facebook posts coming. I love learning all I can about the latest updates!

Wishing you wisdom and happiness!"

A. Greenwood
Breckinridge, Mo.

I'm not going to pretend this happens with everyone, nor do I deserve all the credit. She deserves the credit for persevering, following the plan, and believing that something else was possible.

There are also some really important takeaways here.

Firstly, the answer wasn't just thyroid replacement hormone. This is the answer for some people, but not for everyone. Especially post partum when things are really in flux and your body is adapting to a new normal.

There are also fillers in thyroid medication that may be problematic for some people.

This case also shows that sometimes the thyroid isn't the direct cause of the problems. Here it was the inflammatory process, the adrenals, and an immune system that was out of balance.

It took some digging and detective work to look elsewhere for solutions, but there were pretty clear indications about where they were. What's also really encouraging about this case is that the changes were sustained over more than a year.

That's a very good sign.

So if you're struggling, and the solution that has been offered to you isn't working, then don't be afraid to dig deeper and look for solutions in other systems of the body.

Chapter Fifteen

The Thyroid & the Adrenals

How the Adrenals & the Thyroid Interact

Thyroxine Treatment Can Cause Adrenal Problems

One of the things that doctors rarely discuss is that treatment with T4, like Synthroid or Levothyroxine, can have a major impact on the adrenals.

If someone has adrenal insufficiency, then they are at risk for thyroxine making the problem worse!

Even if the adrenal insufficiency is mild to moderate, it may have an effect on thyroid conversion, tissue uptake, and thyroid response. And not in a good way.

If the T4 to T3 conversion doesn't happen as it should, the body can become overloaded with unused T4.

If it is converted, but the T3 cannot enter the cell walls due to adrenal insufficiency or iron deficiency, the T3 cannot be used, and may pool or build up in the blood.

When this happens, you may suddenly feel all the hyper symptoms like heart palpitations, insomnia, nervousness, etc. This is one of the reasons why some Hashimoto's people may experience hyper to hypo cycles.

In many cases, T4 and TSH blood tests will appear normal, but the patient will feel really lousy.

If a doctor raises the thyroxine dose in this situation, things may become worse. How bad depends on the degree of adrenal insufficiency.

Symptoms may include all the symptoms mentioned above.

Here's what is written on the warning label for Synthroid, but is true of all synthetic T4 drugs.

"Patients with concomitant adrenal insufficiency should be treated with replacement glucocorticoids prior to initiation of treatment with levothyroxine sodium.

Failure to do so may precipitate an acute adrenal crisis when thyroid hormone therapy is initiated, due to increased metabolic clearance of glucocorticoids by thyroid hormone."

What this means, in plain English, is that in cases of hypothyroidism, the adrenals need to be evaluated before putting patients on thyroid replacement hormone.

How many people with Hashimoto's and hypothyroidism do you think have adrenal insufficiency?

I put this question to my <u>Facebook support group</u> and 100% of the 85 respondents with Hashimoto's said they had most of the symptoms of adrenal insufficiency mentioned in the list I posted above.

Granted, that's not a scientific study, but it certainly is emblematic of this problem.

Have you ever heard of a doctor checking for this prior to beginning treatment?

It's not very common, believe you me. Many doctors dismiss adrenal insufficiency as one of those make believe disorders.

The Flip Side

The other side of this is the many ways that adrenal stress can cause hypothyroidism.

As we discussed above, it affects with the HPA axis and this, in turn, disrupts the HPT (hypothamus-pituitary-thyroid) axis. Communication gets all garbled all around.

And we all know how important good communication is. Especially when you have a super-complicated body to run.

Adrenal Stress Can Lead to Autoimmunity

The inside of the body has three main barriers, the blood-brain barrier, the digestive tract and the lungs.

These barriers prevent the bad guys from getting into the bloodstream and the brain. As we saw in the chapter on leaky gut, when they break down, a whole cascade of trouble can follow.

Cortisol can be one of the factors that leads to this breakdown of these barriers and it can impact immune function in a couple of different ways. Since cortisol calms the immune system, too title cortisol can lead to too much immune stimulation and an over-aggressive immune reaction.

And too much cortisol can weaken the immune system and make it harder for you to defend yourself against infections. This immune system suppression can lead to further breakdown of the intestinal lining because the immune system in the get is not strong enough to defend itself.

When the barrier systems break down, proteins, bacteria, viruses, fungi and other large particles can leak into the bloodstream or the brain where they don't belong. Over time, this positive feedback loop repeats over and over again and the immune system is put on high alert.

This is the process that leads to allergies, sensitivities, intolerances and eventually to autoimmune diseases like Hashimoto's.

Adrenal Stress Leads to Thyroid Hormone Resistance

Thyroid hormone doesn't work in the body if it can't turn on receptors inside of cells in the body.

One factor that makes these receptors less sensitive is the systemic inflammation that is at the root of Hashimoto's. The immune proteins that we looked at in the chapters on the metal element are responsible for this.

This inflammation blocks thyroid hormone from getting into the cells and it clogs the receptors.

It's like thyroid hormone is a little dog barking outside the door of the cell and the inflammation is making so much noise that the cell can't hear it. And it just gets ignored.

This is another cause of "functional hypothyroidism". In this situation, the person may be taking thyroid hormone medication, but they still have all the hypothyroid symptoms. And raising the dose doesn't help or only helps temporarily because the problem isn't too little thyroid hormone, it's unresponsive thyroid hormone receptors.

And the blood tests for these patients may look perfect; TSH, T3 and T4 can all be normal.

Adrenal Stress Reduces Conversion of T4 to T3

As we learned in the chapters on the thyroid, 93% of the hormone produced in the thyroid gland is T4. But T4 must be converted into T3 before it can be used by the cells in the body.

The immune proteins that cause receptor problems can also affect conversion of T4 to T3. This transformation is made possible by an enzyme called 5 alpha deiodinase. This happens in the liver, the gut and in the peripheral tissues of the body.

Some of the TH-1 and TH-2 proteins (i.e., IL-6, TNF-alpha and IL-1) that we looked at earlier have been shown to suppress thyroid hormone conversion. In fact, studies have shown that IL-6 (which is often found in abdominal fat) can reduce T3. There's a direct link, so as IL-6 levels go up, T3 levels go down.

The immune cells mentioned above can make T3 levels go down and reverse T3 levels go up. Reverse T3 is a form of T3 that is inactive, it doesn't work on the cells of the body.

So, as you can see, this one process can lead to thyroid receptors not working properly, and thyroid hormone not getting converted and the result is that it doesn't work the way it should.

Adrenal Stress Can Also Cause Hormonal Imbalances

And if that wasn't enough, cortisol also has a powerful effect on the liver. High cortisol caused by chronic stress impairs liver function by slowing down certain pathways.

This cans prevent the liver from being able to clear out certain hormones, like estrogen. Estrogen causes more thyroid binding globulin (TBG) to be produced in the body. TBG are proteins that attach to thyroid hormone. It's kind of like a subway train that shuttles thyroid hormone through the blood.

When thyroid hormone is catching a ride with thyroid binding globulin, it is inactive, which means it doesn't work. It has to get off the train and be freed before it can activate receptors on the cells. (These are the free-fraction thyroid hormones that you see on lab tests: such as free T3 and Free T4)

When TBG levels are high, there are fewer free thyroid hormones. You can see this on a lab test as low T3 Uptake and low free T3 or free T4.

What To Do?

Here's the thing. With Hashimoto's we are constantly under a great deal of physiological stress. You can't just take something for the adrenals and hope for the best. You can't just treat this one child.

Adrenal stress has many causes. These include: anemias, blood sugar imbalances, gut inflammation, food intolerances (like gluten), vitamin, nutrient and essential fatty acid deficiencies, environmental toxins, chronic emotional and psychological stress.

Sound familiar?

These are also all the things that make Hashimoto's worse
.
You can't ignore them or pretend like they aren't there like so many doctors do. We have to deal with all of them.

All of them. Half measures don't lead to half results, they often lead to no results.

When they exist, these conditions must be addressed or any attempt to support the adrenals directly will either fail or be only partially successful.

This is so much more than a thyroid problem.

It's a multi-system problem.

We'll cover what to do for your adrenals in a moment.

Alright, wow, we covered a ton there.

Quick Recap

The adrenals are extremely important. They must be properly assessed and treated.

Five things that can lead to hypothyroidism that are caused by stress and the adrenals are:

1. Disruption of the HPA axis. The queen of mean ruins everybody's evening.

2. Compromised conversion of T4 to T3.

3. Autoimmunity.

4. Thyroid hormone resistance.

5. Hormone imbalances.

It's all connected, it's not linear, and it's not a one-size-fits-all solution. You can do it, but only if you tackle all of these contributing factors. And it might just take more than reading this book to do it.

That's a lot to take in! Let's just sit in silence for the next few minutes and rest. Ohmmmmmm.

HASHIMOMENT:
KNOW YOUR LIMITATIONS

*When we have Hashimoto's,
we have to understand our limitations.*

*Sometimes, you just need to take a seat and rest.
When making plans, make sure to give yourself an
opportunity to do less if you need to.*

Sometimes it's okay to say "No."

It will all get done in due time.

Chapter Sixteen

The Chinese Medicine View
of the Water Element

The Water Element

The Chinese medical view of the kidney includes two completely different sets of characteristics.

The yin organ of the water element is the kidney, but the kidneys themselves have two aspects. There is kidney yin and kidney yang.

Each of the kidneys has a slightly different shape and slightly different location in our body. They aren't exactly symmetrical.

That may be one possible explanation why the ancient Chinese had different ways of looking at them. Kidney yin is the organ itself, and kidney yang, in my opinion, sounds like the endocrine system. And the various adrenal hormones can also be viewed as yin and yang. Cortisol and DHEA are more yin, norepinephrine and epinephrine are more yang.

The Water element's yang organ is the urinary bladder, which doesn't do a lot in western physiology but in Chinese medical physiology, the urinary bladder channel is hugely important.

It can be used to treat all the major organs of the body and to treat a host of psychological and emotional conditions. It taps into every major nerve coming out of the spinal cord (you can see it depicted in the graphic at the beginning of the chapter, the dots are the urinary bladder channel).

The tissue related to the kidneys is the bones, and makes sense, given what we know about the kidneys' role in activating Vitamin D for bone growth and bone remodeling.

The sense organ is the ear and, in fact, in the developing fetus the ears and the kidneys both develop in the fifth to eighth week of pregnancy.

The Water element's negative emotion is fear, and this is interesting because the stress response is all about fear. That's what drives fight or flight—fear.

The kidneys are thought to be responsible for will or aspiration. They store refined substances known as jing, which is linked to reproduction and inherited traits. The ancient Chinese identified the concept of DNA and genes, which is what jing embodies.

Fear in the kidneys is associated with cold, producing chills and shivering. This has a physiological basis in that cold stimulates the adrenal glands and, in turn, produces the stress reactions of fear, fright, shock, and alarm.

The hormones that correlate to the kidney yang are the adrenaline, epinephrine, a little bit of dopamine, and some endogenous opiates.

These hormones, as we have discussed, come from the medulla and respond to stimuli from the nervous system.

What do these yang hormones do? Give you yang energy! They increase metabolism, heart rate, blood pressure, blood flow to the legs, lung function, and metabolic functions in the liver.

The kidney yin aspect of the adrenals is the adrenal cortex and the corticosteroids that influence blood sugar and mineral metabolism. Sex hormones are also released under the influence of ACTH.

Aldosterone has a role in sodium, potassium, and water balance. Cortisol is anti-inflammatory, and the Chinese identified cortisol imbalances as "false heat" or an improper inflammatory condition.

This is found in kidney yin deficiency. Interestingly, cortisol is also responsible for the anti-inflammatory effects of acupuncture. From a spiritual and emotional level, the water element has profound influence.

Water Is the Highest Form of Goodness

The Taoists hold water in very high esteem.

In Chapter 8 of the *Tao The Ching* water is spoken of "The highest form of goodness is like water. Water knows how to benefit all things without striving with them. It stays in places loathed by all men. Therefore it comes near the Tao."

So the irony of the Water element is that, at its heart, it teaches us that true power comes from wisdom, which results in the cultivation of our resources.

Resources are our energy, our time, our emotions, all of that. Right? If you get over-extended, then you deplete those resources

But this chronic reaction to fear, the chronic stress response, drives the kidneys and bladder officials to either over- or under-utilize willpower to control the use of our resources.

If we are reckless with the resources that we have, ambition may push us to exhaustion as we try to make our way in the world. With every new project we complete, the feelings of success and accomplishment are fleeting, and fear shows up again and we're off to the next project.

Have you ever experienced that? Jeez, I sure have. And where does it get us? Burnt out.

Remember when I sighted that statistic about 80 percent of people with autoimmune disease had experienced some very stressful event prior to its onset?

On the other hand, if we are very conservative with our resources, we may get frozen by this fear and do very little. Every project is potentially rewarding, but then the fear kicks in and we pull back and stop it midstream.

So the wisdom inherent in the Water element teaches us how to balance these two extremes so we don't get burnt out, and so we don't get paralyzed by fear into inactivity. There has got to be a happy medium.

The bladder is involved in the storage and usage of things we acquire during our lives, such as the experiences, the wisdom, and what else we collect along the way.

So another way of understanding the resources that the kidneys help us use and save is the idea of our inherited constitution. This is called jing, and really relates to DNA, but also to our inherited emotional and spiritual essence.

Jing Is a Metaphor for Our Own Well

Jing is the water in our well. Jing is distributed to all the other yin organs by the kidneys. Jing also stores all of our life's potential—our destiny—in a sense. This potential must be conserved and used wisely over the course of our lives as our destiny unfolds.

The general idea is to draw only as much as you need for the task at hand and save the rest. You want to live off the interest of what you collect along the way and do your best to save your inheritance.

The life issues of those of us with problems involving this yang energy revolve around the general theme of utilizing our resources appropriately.

Hashimoto's involves a deficiency of yang. We see this in various endocrine glands: the adrenals, the pancreas, the thyroid, and the pituitary.

So when our kidney energy is not functioning harmoniously, we overspend, over work, over play, just over do it in general.

In his book, *Nourishing Destiny*, Lonnie Jarrett tells a great story that sums this concept up beautifully. I've paraphrased and embellished it a bit here.

There's a beggar who lives on the street in a marketplace in ancient China. And a genie sees him and decides to help him.

So he approaches the beggar and asks, "How much money would be enough to help a poor man?" The beggar says 500 hundred yuan, (that's the currency.) Of course, after a few days the money is spent and the beggar is back on the street sleeping in the marketplace.

So the genie sees him again and asks, "How much money would be enough to help you?" The beggar thinks about it, revises his calculation and says "10, 000 yuan".

This time he is able to buy a small house and hire servants. But over time, he doesn't save his money. He spends it here, there and everywhere and loses it all and winds up back at the marketplace, sleeping in the street.

So the genie approaches him a third time and the beggar sees him and reflects on his previous 2 experiences and says "100,000 yuan will last me for a lifetime, I know it."

So now, he's a little more savvy, he buys nice clothes, gets married, has a family. And this is a lot of money in those days. So he has prestige and people notice and he gets appointed to high ranking position in the court.

But, he is who he is. And he hasn't learned the fundamental lesson from the water element. So he lives large and spends big and because of his excessive lifestyle and some bad investments, he loses it all again and descends into misery, winding up on the street sleeping in the marketplace.

The genie sees him and takes pity and decides to help him one last time. The beggar sees the genie walking towards him and gets up and runs for the hills.

So that's the lesson of the water element, we must learn how to care for and save what we are given. That is really key and may be the most important lesson of all of this entire book.

If we want to heal our Hashimoto's this idea of not depleting what we have is hugely important. And what does that mean in real life?

Just like we need to take the sugar balance problem seriously, we really need to take the impact of stress on our bodies, minds and souls seriously. Living that type A, hard running lifestyle will, over time, result in you squandering your reserves. There is no question about it.

Ok, the water element. Let's rest. Take a little break to think about this in our own lives and when we come back we'll look at how the bladder energy and spirit figures into this.

Savings In The Bank

So we looked at the kidney's role in preserving our inheritance. Let's take a look at the bladder's role in saving and using what we collect along the way.

According to the *Nei Jing*, the bladder is responsible for regions of the body, it stores the body fluids.

As we have seen with other yang partners to the yin organ, the function of the yang organ is to assist the yin partner and kind of be a conduit to the outside world.

So with the kidneys, the spirit of the kidneys is the will. When the kidney and the bladder are working together harmoniously, wisdom is manifest in everything you do.

The bladder orchestrates the inheritance, your natural talents and abilities and genetic predisposition and like a good accountant it helps you manage what your life brings you.

The money, the experiences, the relationships, etc. It's like a reservoir. A reservoir needs to be able to hold water without losing it and it needs to be able to expand when there's lots of rain and it provides water when you need it.

The healthy function of the bladder is to empower us to assess adequately both the quantity and quality of our reserves. Like the will, the bladder must guide us to spend our resources the right way. Not to just blow your savings impulsively.

So, when the water element is out of balance, fear rules. Chronic stress takes over. Even though no immediate threat is there, we live in a constant state that we won't have enough or that we are going to lose what we do have, etc.

This causes the separation of the heart and the mind and it prevents the bladder from accessing that innate wisdom. Without that wisdom, you lose perspective.

This is why anxiety is a very common symptom of adrenal problems. Fear takes over and it's out of context and its there even when there is no real threat.

When this happens the kidney can't communicate with the outside world and it becomes secretive and paranoid. Fear is the result.

228

Another analogy regarding the bladder is that this is like a person driving a car and and they see the gas light turn on, but then they see a sign that says next gas station is in 10 miles. Have you ever done that?

So you start asking yourself:

"Is it really empty? I heard they make it a lot higher so you can go a long way on empty." And "Why didn't I fill up the darn tank when I had the chance?"

And if you're in the next car, this car looks fine. You don't see all this internal chatter or anxiety. You don't see that the reserves are severely depleted.

Right? This person is driving fast because they are freaking out, not because they're just loving their car.

This happens when you have an urgent need to pee, too. You get nervous and anxious, can't focus on other stuff, you got to go. That overstimulation feeling is common with the bladder, in general.

> *The feeling of being over stimulated is also very common with Hashimoto's.*
> *We are under so much physiological stress all the time, that it's really easy to to get over stimulated.*

Remember when I spoke about the bladder channel running down the back and accessing the virtually the entire nervous system via the spinal cord?

That's a bladder problem, overstimulation of the nervous system.

Quick Recap

Ok, let's recap.

The water element and the kidneys are about our natural wisdom, and our will.

The yin organ is the kidney, the yang organ is the bladder. The adrenals are the endocrine gland and they also have their own yin and yang character.

Fear is the dominant emotional of the water element. And when fear drives your life you suffer the consequences, eventually you burn out.

When we looked at how many ways the adrenals and stress can lead to problems with Hashimoto's and our health, that's what this is all about.

So we need to heal the water element. We need to get a handle on our fears and conserve our resources so we have enough in the tank when we need it.

We need to calm our nervous systems and support the adrenals. Let's take a look at some things that do just that.

There are 3 basic stages of adrenal fatigue and exhaustion.

In this final part of the chapter, we will look at those and look at some testing for the adrenals.

But before we get there, let's look at a few things that you can do to support your adrenals and help heal them.

How to Support and Heal Your Adrenals

Numero Uno: Avoid stimulants, especially the super caffeinated sugar based coffee and energy drinks. These are the physiological equivalent of running up credit card debt and putting nothing in your bank account.

Talk about emptying your reserves, you will definitely need a bail out after these. These drinks do nothing for you nutritionally. They destroy your adrenals and quickly rob you of any energetic savings you may have.

Have a little green tea if you need a pick me up. Other things to avoid include: ephedra, caffeine, guarana, kola nut and prescription stimulants like Adderall, Ritalin, Concerta and that new super expensive diet drug Qsymia or Phentermine.

Balance Your Blood Sugar

To minimize stress on the adrenal system, and ensure maximum energy, you should consider a low-glycemic (low-sugar) diet, consisting of sufficient protein and fat, low-glycemic carbohydrates, eaten in smaller, more frequent meals throughout the day.

This is precisely why I advocate the Autoimmune Paleo diet that we spoke about in the previous chapter.

Practice stress management and relaxation techniques: meditation, yoga, qi gong etc.

Also, make sure you have at least one day a week where you do nothing. I mean nothing. Schedule down time. Many people have lives that are so busy that even there time off is over loaded. I was one of those people. Trust me, you can't sustain it.

Have fun, laugh and make pleasure a regular part of your life. Have fun people! We need to laugh.

Avoid dietary causes of inflammation. These drain your adrenals. (refined flours, high-fructose corn syrup and industrial seed oils in particular). You can control what you put in your mouth.

Ensure adequate intake of DHA & EPA. These are omega 3 fatty acids, and they're very beneficial for the adrenal glands. Natural sources include: fish oil, flax seed oil, krill oil, hemp seed oil, etc.

Another important thing that can undermine adrenal health is toxicity issues. If you are having an immune reaction to environmental toxins, like heavy metals, mold or chemicals, and you don't work on these, then you won't get anywhere with your adrenals.

Something else that can be beneficial for the adrenals and kidneys are a group of herbs that may be helpful are herbs called adaptogens: in the 1940's a Soviet scientist named Dr. Nikolai Lazarev coined the phrase adaptogen and defined these botanicals as "an agent that reassess the body's ability to resist stress by countering undesired stressors, whether physical, chemical, emotional or biological."

These herbs have been used for hundreds of years in Chinese medicine. The beauty of these herbs from a Chinese medical perspective is that they can be combined into powerful adaptogenic formulae for healing the adrenals and helping the body adapt to stress.

Adaptogens are thought to work on normalizing the hypothalmic-pituitary-adrenal (HPA) axis. I have provided a more complete list in the following chapter.

I thought maybe we'd take a look at one adaptogenic herb and examine it's pharmacology, so you can see an example of how this works.

This herb is called **Ci Wu Jia** in Chinese, the botanical name is **Eleuthrococcus senticosus**. It is traditionally a spleen and kidney tonic and is used for low back and knee pain and physical weakness, insomnia and anorexia.

Pharmacologically it does a lot:

It is a mild sedative for the central nervous system - so it's calming.

It increases endurance and lessens fatigue - so it can give you energy in a nutritious way, unlike an energy drink.

It protects the body from radiation.

It enhances immune function in a number of different ways.

It is anti-cancer.

It is anti-inflammatory.

It increases coronary blood flow.

It is anti-bacterial.

And in cases of low resistance or extra demand on physical strength and mental work such as high altitude flying, long distance sailing, working in high or low temperature or in deep water (all very stressful environments) this herb was found to increase physical strength, improve mental power and increase vision, color vision and hearing.

Wow! Do you think that might be beneficial for adrenal fatigue or stress? Yes, indeed.

Recap: Healing the Water Element

The water element. The kidney is yin, the urinary bladder is yang. The adrenals have both yin and yang aspects.

The negative emotion of the water element is fear. We must learn to not let fear control us or dictate our decisions and manipulate our will.

This can block us from our innate wisdom, separate our hearts from our minds and force us to lose our way.

Some keys to healing the adrenals are:

1. Avoiding stimulants.

2. Balancing blood sugar.

3. Practicing stress management. Not just thinking about it actually doing things like meditation, yoga, qi gong, taking days off, having down time, etc.

5. Avoiding dietary causes of inflammation. Gut infections, and inflammation are chronic adrenal stressors all by themselves.

6. Making sure we're getting enough omega 3's in our diet.

7. And adding adaptogenic herbs to our mix of supplements.

Chapter Seventeen

Using the A.P.A.R.T. System to Heal the Water Element

The A.P.A.R.T. System

1. A = Ask and Asses

Open your journal again and look for symptoms of problems with the Water Element. Note what they are, then create a plan for addressing them. After that, you must act on your plan. Follow through and do what you have planned.

After that take inventory of what you did. Look at what worked and what didn't. Both will provide valuable information.

Double down on what worked, change what didn't. Keep at it.

Winter is an excellent time to heal Water Element issues. But don't wait to deal with stress and heal the adrenals. They are just too important to wait.

Signs and Symptoms of Adrenal Fatigue

Category XI Adrenals-Low Cortisol
Cannot stay asleep
Crave salt
Slow starter in the morning
Afternoon fatigue
Dizziness when standing up quickly
Afternoon headaches
Headaches with exertion or stress
Weak nails

Category XII Adrenals-High Cortisol
Cannot fall asleep
Perspire easily
Under high amount of stress
Weight gain when under stress
Wake up tired even after 6 or more hours of sleep
Excessive perspiration or perspiration with little or no activity

Kidney Symptoms Caused by Hypothyroidism

The kidneys are a perfect place to see how the different systems of the body are impacted by hypothyroidism and Hashimoto's:

Hypothyroidism can cause:

* Less blood flow to the kidneys

(This can cause creatinine to build up and not be excreted. Creatinine is a chemical waste molecule that is generated from muscle metabolism.)

* **Increased amounts of uric acid.** 20-30% of gout patients have hypothyroidism. This is often linked with higher levels of creatinine.

* **High blood pressure.** According to one study, up to 40% of hypothyroid patients had high blood pressure.

The kidneys fail to filter waste products from your body properly when your pressure is low, and "angiotensin" is produced, which raises your blood pressure.

Also, a rise in cortisol from your adrenals can raise your blood pressure.

Hypothyroidism can also cause edema.

You can see this swelling under the eyes, or as mild swelling of the hands and feet.

This is caused by several things: decreased kidney function, capillaries becoming more permeable-, poor lymphatic drainage and salt and water retention by the kidneys.

These changes, in turn can lead to some serious problems with both the heart and kidneys.

General Symptoms of Kidney Imbalance from a TCM point of View

All bone problems, especially those of the knees, lower back, and teeth
Back pain, especially in the area of the kidneys, which are located midway down the back just below the lower rib cage.
Hearing loss and ear infections and diseases
Head-hair problems- hair loss, split ends, premature graying
Any urinary, reproductive and/or sexual issues
Poor growth and development
Excessive fear and insecurity
Premature graying of the hair

Testing the Adrenals

In this last section I'd like to take a look at some testing we can do for the adrenals and also to talk about the 3 stages of adrenal burnout.

Ok, so like virtually everything in our body, things don't usually happen overnight. They develop over time and progress from ok, to sort of bad to really bad if you do't do anything to stop that progression.

We saw this with the progression to type 2 diabetes. It goes from dysglycemia to insulin resistance to metabolic syndrome to full blown diabetes.

The same is true with autoimmune disease. It goes from silent autoimmunity to reactive autoimmunity to full blown autoimmune disease.

The adrenals are no exception. Adrenal problems also go through a progression as well.

It looks like this:

3 Stages of Adrenal Dysfunction

1. Alarm reaction: This happens in normal life. The adrenal glands become hyperactive to increase cortisol levels to adapt to the demands of stress.

2. The second stage is the Resistance stage: This occurs in response to prolonged stress as the body steals pregnenolone from cholesterol to make cortisol- we spoke about this- the pregnenolone steal.

When this happens, hormonal imbalances arise because there isn't enough cholesterol to use them. It can cause PMS, infertility, male menopause, and polycystic ovarian syndrome (PCOS).

3. The third stage is the Exhaustion stage: At the point the adrenals are saying "Uncle" and they can no longer adapt to stress.

The cofactors need to make cortisol become depleted and cortisol levels drop too low. Because the adrenals no longer produce sufficient cortisol, the pregnenolone steal cycle also stops.

There are a few tests that you can do at home and I've included these in the supplemental materials.

How to Test your Adrenals at Home

Basically, let me give you a quick run down of what they are.

The first is to test your blood pressure in 2 different positions: sitiing or lying down and standing.

Firstly, Take and compare two blood pressure readings—one while lying down or sitting and one while standing. Rest for five minutes in a relaxed position before taking the reading.

Stand up and immediately check your blood pressure again. If the blood pressure is **lower** after standing, then you may have reduced adrenal gland function, and more specifically, an aldosterone issue–(Aldosterone is an adrenal hormone and hypothyroidism can lead to low levels of aldostrone in the blood.)

(Normal adrenal function will elevate your BP on the standing reading in order to push blood to the brain.)

It's also a good idea to do this test both in the morning and in the evening, becasue you can appear normal one time, and not another.

A Second Adrenal Test

The second test you can do is to check your pupils. This is called the **Pupil Test** and it also tests levels of aldosterone,.

You need to be in a dark room with a mirror. From the side (not the front), shine a bright light like a flashlight or penlight towards your pupils and hold it for about a minute. Carefully observe what happens to your pupil.

With healthy adrenals (and specifically, healthy levels of aldosterone),your pupils will constrict, and will stay small the entire time you shine the light from the side.

The light causes them to constrict, it's a natural response to having light shone in your eye.

In adrenal fatigue, the pupil will get small, but within 30 seconds, it will soon get larger again again or obviously start to flutter as it tries to stay small.

Why does this happen?

Because when you have adrenal insufficiency you can also have low aldosterone, which can cause an imbalance in sodium and potassium (too little sodium and too much potassium).

This imbalance is what causes the sphincter muscles of your eye to be weak and to dilate in response to light.

So the fluttering struggle to keep the pupil small may mean you have adrenal challenges.

Adrenal Lab Test

In terms of laboratory tests, by far the best one is ASI or Adrenal Salivary Index. This provides the most accurate, useful and comprehensive test for the adrenals.

One important thing to understand about this test. And this is true of a number of different tests. The most important test is the second or even third test.

One test is useless, because we are establishing a baseline and then we are going to take action. And we need to know if what we are doing is helping.

The second and third tests give us that information. We must always reassess and readjust.

And the adrenals generally respond to treatment pretty well. If they don't you need to look for something deeper. A parasite or heavy metal toxicity, a chronic viral infection or some food intolerance.

Sometimes you have to be a detective and rule out these infections or intolerances.

The ASI tells us how a person's adrenals are working throughout the day. Its a 24 hour test. Cortisol is secreted in a specific pattern over a 24 hour day and by measuring saliva at different intervals throughout the day, we can chart the cortisol levels.

Being in a chronic state of alarm or prolonged stress will mess with this rhythm. One example of this is people who are night owls, or have trouble falling, staying asleep or they wake up really tired after getting enough sleep. Their rhythm has been disrupted.

The ASI shows abnormalities in this circadian rhythm, charts key hormone levels and pinpoints where problems arise along the way. It can be a really valuable test.

You can learn more about herbs and nutritional support for each stage of adrenal dysfunction in the next section.

Ok, let's wrap it up here. We covered an awful lot in this section.

Adrenal Testing Recap

Some of the tests that you can do for the adrenals are:

1. The blood pressure test. Take 2 measurements, one seated or lying downand one standing. Compare them. If there is a big difference, this may pointto adrenal problems.

2. The pupil test. Point a light at your pupils. Watch it constrict, then watch it return to normal. If it gets small and then quickly goes back to normal or flutters, then this is positive for adrenal issues.

3. Lastly, the best laboratory test is the ASI or Adrenal Salivary Index. This takes multiple saliva tests throughout the day and tracks your circadian rhythm. It can be very helpful, not only for identifying the problem but also for tracking your progress in fixing it.

Awesome! The water element. The kidneys, the bladder , the adrenals. Fear and loathing in your body.

We have to deal with stress. It can be very destructive and it does real damage. It is something we really have to take seriously.

If we want to heal out Hashimoto's, we absolutely have to heal our adrenals. And the reality is that this whole process of healing these multiple systems is, without question going to take longer than it takes you to read this book.

I am teaching you about what is going on. Correcting it takes time, patience, vigilance and devotion.

But it is so worth it, people.

Alright, I love this stuff. Its so fascinating.

2. P = Prioritize and Plan

Not everything has the same level importance. This is what 80/20 teaches us. Some things are having more of an impact than others. Figure out which they are (the positive feedback loops) and then make a plan to fix them.

What does that mean when it comes to the Water Element? Check kidney and adrenal function. Adrenal health is very important if you are taking thyroid replacement hormone.

Remember the warning label for Synthroid that we looked at earlier in the chapter. Clearly, evaluating and treating the adrenals, if necessary, is a major priority.

3. A = Act and Adapt

Water: Kidneys, Urinary Bladder and Adrenals

Foods:

-Foods which nurture Kidney Yin- string bean, black bean, mung bean and its sprouts, kidney bean, most other beans, kuzu root, watermelon and other melons, blackberry, muleberry, blueberry, huckleberry, water chestnut, seaweed, spirulina, chlorella, black sesame seed, sardine, crab, clan, eggs, pork

-Kidney Yang deficiency- Cloves, black peppercorn, ginger, cinnamon bark, walnuts, black bean, onion family, quinoa, chicken, lamb, trout, and salmon

-Treating damp heat in bladder (bladder infections)- broth ingredients can be chosen from- aduki beans, lima beans, celery, carrots, winter squash, asparagus, mushrooms and other vegetables that are not warming, Recommended fruit- lemon(diluted juice), cranberry(diluted juice or tablets), huckleberries

-Building jing-micro-algea, fish, liver, kidney, brain, bone and its marrow, human placenta, and cereal grass, , chicken and mussle

Herbs/Supplements:

-Herbs which nurture kidney yin- marshmallow root, prepared rehmannia root, mandarin, asparagus root, aloe vera gel, silver colloid

-Deficient kidney qi- rose hips, oyster shell, clam shell, schisandra fruit, raspberry, blackberry leaves, and gravel root

-Treating damp heat in bladder (bladder infections)- beneficial herbal teas- uva ursi, dandelion leaf, plantain leaf, pipsissewa, flax seed and watermelon seed

-Building jing- nettle, royal jelly, and bee pollen, dodder seeds, deer antler, mandarin, tortoise shell

Adaptogenic Herbs:

There are quite a few herbs that have adaptogenic properties, meaning that they help your body apt to stress.

But as with everything, there is a risk/benefit analysis that must be done with them, especially when autoimmunity is involved. You must be cautious about stimulating the immune system when taking adaptogenic herbs.

Here's a list of herbs that can be helpful, it may be best to introduce them one at a time rather than in a mixed formula. That way, if you have a reaction, you'll know which herb was responsible:

Acanthopanax
American gensing
Ashwaghanda (this plant is a nightshade and may cause a reaction)
Cordyceps
Codonopsis
Eleuthrococcus
He shou wu (also excellent for helping promote hair growth)
Holy Basil
Jiaogulan (also excellent for reducing cholesterol)
Licorice
Maca
Panax gensing
Rhodiola
Schizandra

Herbs that influence ACTH: ACTH is to the adrenals what TSH is to the thyroid. It regulates cortisol production. High ACTH may mean the adrenals aren't producing enough cortisol. Low ACTH may mean the pituitary isn't producing enough adrenals hormones.

ACTH Increasing:

Ginko
Panax ginseng

Tripterygium

ACTH Reducing:

Acanthopanax
Hypercium
Licorice

Suggestions for Different Stages of Adrenal fatigue/Exhaustion

1. Alarm Stage:

Balance blood sugar and support healthy response to insulin resistance: alpha lipoic acid, biotin, chromium, gynemma sylvestre, inositol, magnesium, zinc

Adaptogens: See above

Essential fatty acids: fish oil, evening primrose oil

2. Resistance Stage:

Balance blood sugar and support healthy response to insulin resistance: alpha lipoic acid, biotin, chromium, gynemma sylvestre, inositol, magnesium, zinc

Adaptogens: See above

Essential fatty acids: fish oil, evening primrose oil

Add licorice, and B vitamins (see food sources below)

3. Adrenal Exhaustion:

Chromium, adrenal, pancreas glands, choline bitartrate, co-enzyme Q 10, inositol, rubidium chelate, vanadium.

Adaptogens: See above

Essential fatty acids: fish oil, evening primrose oil

Add licorice, and B vitamins (see food sources below)

In cases of extreme exhaustion, consider consult a physician or practitioner. You may benefit by adding pregnenolone and DHEA..

Common Issues

Bladder Infection - broth ingredients can be chosen from- aduki beans, lima beans, celery, carrots, winter squash, asparagus, mushrooms and other vegetables that are not warming, Recommended fruit- lemon(diluted juice), cranberry(diluted juice or tablets), huckleberries

Chronic Bladder Infection: Watermelon, pears, carrots, celery, cornsilk, squash, oranges, cantaloupe, grapes, strawberries, lotus root, loquats, plenty of water, and in general cooling, diuretic foods (see edema below)

Edema- (swelling and water retention) ginger skin, winter melon, winter melon skin, squash, apples, mulberries, peaches, tangerines, coconuts, seaweeds, fish, celery, green onions, garlic, bamboo shoots, spinach, water chestnuts, carrots, watermelon, beef

Here are some food sources of B Vitamins.

VITAMIN B1: rice bran, pinto bean, peas, millet, lentils, almonds, turnip greens, collard greens, kale, asparagus

VITAMIN B2: salmon, trout, cod, mackerel, perch, oysters, mushrooms, almonds, hijiki

VITAMIN B3: rice bran, red pepper, wild rice, kelp, sesame seed, peaches, brown rice, mushrooms, barley, almonds, apricot

VITAMIN B5 (PANTOTHENIC ACID): beef, chicken, salmon, mackerel, sardines, barley, rice, avocado, plums, raisins, almonds, dates

VITAMIN B6: banana, barley, brewer's yeast, molasses, brown rice, liver, beef, cabbage, carrots, potato, yams

VITAMIN B12: beef liver, beef kidney, ham, sole, scallops, eggs, oats, pickles, amasake, algae, spirulina and chlorella, brewer's yeast

FOLIC ACID: liver, asparagus, lima beans, spinach, swiss chard, kale, cabbage, sweet corn

An Excellent Kidney Cleanse

Here is a simple kidney cleansing formula that is effective for cleansing the kidneys and dissolving kidney stones.

1 quart pure apple juice (must be organic)
2 ounces hydrangea root (chopped)

Soak hydrangea root in the juice for 12 hours. Put the juice and root on the stove and bring to a boil. Slowly simmer for 30 minutes. Let cool, strain our hydrangea root and bottle. Keep juice in the refrigerator. Drink a cupful 3 to 4 times per day for 3 to 7 days.

Note: Hydrangea root can be purchased whole at most health food stores. It has been used by both Western and Chinese herbalists. It promotes detoxification and clears dampness; dissolves deposits and promotes urination and has also been used to clear damp heat and reduce infections.

It is a gentle, yet effective remedy. **However, it should not be taken for a prolonged period of time and if you have kidney or liver problems you should consult a licensed herbalist before using.**

Also, it is a mild diuretic, so if you are taking diuretics or blood pressure medication you should also consult your doctor. It is also not recommended for pregnant or nursing women.

It can be obtained as a tincture, which is the herb in liquid extract form. If you want to use this form, then modify the formula by filling a cup with apple juice and adding 20-30 drops of hydrangea tincture. Drink warm or cold.

Qi Gong Exercise for the Water Element
Bending for Health

Bending for health

Purpose and Effect: The mind-set during this exercise is that you are gathering the highest-quality energy from heaven and earth as you move. As you gather the best of the best energy, you are nurturing your personal Qi.

The waist and abdominal area are the focus in this exercise. The purpose is to stimulate the kidneys, adrenaline glands, and arterial and venous circulation of the lower abdomen.

In Chinese medicine, affecting the kidneys can aid the teeth, hearing, and urinary system, including water-retention problems. Stimulating the adrenal glands can assist both the urinary and respiratory systems. The solar plexus and lumbar nerve plexus area are also exercised and stimulated.

When you lean backward, you are guiding energy up from your feet and out of your head. In more physical terms, leaning forward and backward affect blood flow to the brain. It strengthens the nervous system, adjust overall body metabolism, and improves coordination of the internal organs. This exercise also tones the abdominals, strengths sexual ability, clears your mind, and brightens your vision. It also helps prostate problems in men and reproductive system problems in women.

CAUTION: People with serious illness, especially heart disease or high blood pressure, should do this exercise lightly and should not bend very far forward or backward.

How to Begin: Move your left foot out so feet are little wider than shoulder-width apart.

As you inhale, sweep your hands to your sides and out front, bringing them close to the abdomen across from where your kidneys are, palms facing abdomen (a).

As you exhale, place palms on your kidneys (midback), thumbs to the front, fingers pointing to the back (b). Keeping your legs fairly straight and your knees loose. (Note: People with hand problems may place the hands lower on the back or buttocks to relieve pressure on the wrist and finger joints.)

As you inhale, lengthen your spine and lean backward as far as comfortable (c). Try to stretch and bend back all along the spine. Keep in mind that the goal is to straighten and strengthen the spine.

As you exhale, bend forward as far as possible, allowing your head to hang down in front of your body (d). It is important to keep both the waist and the back muscles as soft and relaxed as possible.

As you inhale, return to a standing position with your palms on your kidneys again, lengthen your spine and look up and over, leaning backward as far as is comfortable (e).

As you exhale, straighten up, sweeping your arms slightly above and in front of your head (f). Then bend forward as far as is comfortable, making your hands sweep downward without any arm muscle movement. If possible, hold your toes (g).

If you can't reach that far, hold your lower legs or knees.

Modifications for Low Stamina: The breathing can be changed so that every step in this exercise involves an inhale and an exhale.

Instead of reaching directly for your toes, place your palms (thumbs on the inside, fingers on the outside) on your thighs and massage downward to your toes (thus massaging the kidney and liver channels).

*Repeat 3 times 1 or 2 times per day.

From The Art of Qi Gong Healing By Master Hong Liu

Want to see a Video demonstration of this? Visit our supplemental area at
https://hashimotos-diet.com/roadmap-to-remission-supplemental/

4. R= Reassess and Readjust

Retest, Reassess and ask all over again. Figure out what worked and what didn't. Double down on what worked and either eliminate or recreate a plan for what didn't.

This an area that is rarely looked at by doctors, but as we saw earlier, Hashimoto's can have far reaching effects on both kidney and heart functions.

It is very important to check kidney function. Order a simple a renal panel and test uric acid levels and electrolytes.

Try some things and reassess.

5. T = Try and Try Again

Keep doing it, keep refining, keep building on the positive results and keep looking for the remaining positive feedback loops that are causing vicious cycles.

The water element is the root of our health. You must continually revisit it.

Chapter Eighteen

Hashimoto's and the Brain

Hashimoto's and hypothyroidism have a profound impact on our brains. This is area that I'm really passionate about.

It's also an area that almost no one talks about or does anything about and I'm totally baffled by this. This is arguably the most important part of our body to talk about and treat.

Several of the most common symptoms of Hashimoto's are brain related. Some of these are obvious such as brain fog and memory loss, others are less so, like depression and neurological disorders which can resemble or develop into Alzheimer's and Parkinson's disease.

Regardless of how obvious they are, all these brain related symptoms are a sign of degeneration of the brain. This is not a good thing.

But before we dive into your brains, let's recap what we've learned in the previous chapters because what we have learned also applies to the brain.

In **Chapter 2** we covered the thyroid and look at how many people are "functionally hypothyroid".

In other words, they are getting enough thyroid hormone, but it's not getting converted properly and/or it isn't getting absorbed into the cells of your body.

There are many reasons for this and we've covered some of them. But the important thing to realize when it comes to the brain is that if thyroid hormone isn't getting properly converted and absorbed, then this might make brain related symptoms worse.

(More on that below.)

Then we looked at the **Metal Element** and immune system. Hashimoto's is, of course an autoimmune disease and this is an area that conventional medicine often just ignores or takes the "let's wait and see" approach.

Which really means, let's wait until 70 to 90 % of that part of your body is destroyed until we do anything.

Common sense tells us that waiting for that much tissue destruction makes no sense.

Well, it turns out that one thing that people with Hashimoto's are at risk for is brain autoimmunity. And this can be really destructive to brain cells.

Finally, we looked at the **Water Element**, the kidneys, the urinary bladder and the adrenals.

And we saw how destructive stress can be for people with Hashimoto's. Because our bodies are under so much physiological stress, we just can't afford additional emotional stress and abnormally stressful events.

They are too costly.

Well, it turns our stress is really costly for brain cells too.

So, let's dive in and have a look at what's going on upstairs.

Thyroid health and brain health are linked from our earliest development in the womb.

Brain and Thyroid Health Start in the Womb

One of the truths that, unfortunately, gets little attention is the impact of a healthy thyroid on the development of a healthy baby, especially a developing baby's brain.

If you have Hashimoto's and you want to get pregnant it is very important for you to test your thyroid early and often.

There is a very real risk of retardation or poor brain development and studies have shown that women who are hypothyroid during pregnancy are 4 times more likely to have a child with autism.

And it is important to realize that if you are taking thyroid replacement hormone that you may need to adjust your dosage in order to ensure that your baby's brain develops properly.

It is also vitally important to be as thyroid healthy as possible *prior* to trying to conceive.

Because this is not only a risk to the baby's brain. One of the leading causes of miscarriage is hypothyroidism. A thyroid workup should be a routine part of any woman's prenatal care. Unfortunately, this is rarely done.

Hypothyroidism Can Cause Problems in a Child's Brain, Too

These risks are not only present in the developing brain of a fetus. Once a child is born, if they have too little thyroid hormone, they can experience issues with learning language and have memory problems.

This may be caused by a number of factors. Some environmental toxins have been shown to negatively impact thyroid hormone production.

In fact, studies have shown that polychlorinated biphenyls (PCBs) alter the expression of thyroid hormone-responsive genes in children's brains.

Hypothyroidism in Adults Can Lead to All Kinds of Cognitive Disorders

In adults, thyroid hormone has been shown to have major influences over virtually every brain activity.

T3 and T4 are involved in the formation of neurons, neuronal migration, axonal and dendritic growth (these are different kinds of nerve fibers), mylenation and more.

Hashimoto's and hypothyroidism can lead to various disorders including lethargy, hyporeflexia and poor motor coordination.

They are also linked to bipolar affective disorders, depression, or loss of cognitive functions, especially in the elderly.

And in the most extreme cases, Hashimoto's can lead to a condition called Hashimoto's Encephalopathy which can cause severe changes in the brain that look very much like the destruction caused by Alzheimer's.

The brain actually loses massive amounts of brain tissue with Hashimoto's Encephalopathy.

Clearly, thyroid hormone has a powerful effect on the brain. And hypothyroidism and brain inflammation can cause serious and lasting damage to the brain.

Brain Fog Is Brain Inflammation

One of the most common symptoms of Hashimoto's is brain fog, that feeling like you are thinking through a haze, like you can't quite focus or concentrate no matter how hard you try.

Brain fog is an indication of inflammation in your brain. Immune cells in the brain, called microglia, are responsible for this.

The immune system in the brain is different than the immune system in the rest of the body. In the body it is much more complex, there are many different parts and they balance and regulate each other.

In your brain, the immune system is simpler. It's like one of those people that has only 2 speeds, sleeping or balls to the wall.

Microglial cells have an extremely hair trigger.

Microglia cell

And they are capable of inflicting major damage. (Think chihuahua with an automatic rifle.) Frighten them or make them mad and there's carnage, everywhere.

These cells are responsible for causing Alzheimer's, Parkinson's, cardiovascular disease and more.

These cells also respond quickly to pathogens and injury, accumulate in regions of degeneration and produce a wide variety of pro-inflammatory molecules.

That's right, they cause inflammation.

Thyroid hormone has a major influence on them. It can help keep them calm and modulate them.

This is why some people with Hashimoto's notice that their brain fog really improves once they are given thyroid hormone.

For many others, this doesn't help at all. If this is the case, there is something else driving the inflammation and the immune attack. (More on this in a moment.)

Fatigue Is Often Brain Based

Another common symptom for people with Hashimoto's is fatigue and in many cases this is being caused by the same brain inflammation.

When these people perform activities that require mental activity, such as reading or driving for long periods of time, they get tired.

Even after they start taking thyroid hormones, they may continue to have these symptoms.

Their brain has less endurance so they get tired when they use their brain for extended periods of time.

If you have fatigue when you read, drive or have long conversations, this is brain-based fatigue.

You cannot get brain endurance back unless you support your brain. At this point it is not simply a thyroid hormone problem anymore.

Other Factors Lead to Brain Degeneration

The thing to realize is that this inflammation and subsequent fatigue may be caused by an autoimmune response and that things that trigger your immune system may be triggering your brain inflammation and degeneration.

Let's take a look at a couple of the usual suspects. One is gluten, the other is leaky gut. Together they equal leaky brain and brain inflammation.

Leaky Gut Can Also Mean Leaky Brain

Microglia cells attacking neurons after being stimulated by foreign particles

A protein found in connection with gluten consumption called **zonulin** (the zipper we discussed earlier) is linked to leaky gut (intestinal permeability) — the very thing that commonly leads to antibody reactions to foods which leads to sensitivities, allergies and even (eventually) things like Hashimoto's.

There is a direct link between inflammation in the gut (commonly generated by irritants such as gluten), microglial activation (as a result of these foreign compounds getting into the bloodstream) and brain degeneration.

Gluten has also been linked to the destruction of cerebellar tissue, and is a known cause of ataxia, which is the loss of control of bodily movements. Researchers M. Hadjivassiliou et al found that a gluten free diet was helpful in treating this condition.

If you have leaky gut, you may also have leaky brain. These same proteins are found in the blood brain barrier. So gluten and other proteins and foreign matter can get into the blood stream and may wind up in your brain.

This is why some people's brain fog doesn't improve with thyroid hormone. It's not just a thyroid hormone problem, other factors are leading to inflammation in the brain.

In order to improve brain fog, you must reduce brain inflammation and heal the barrier systems because when things enter the brain that shouldn't the microglia respond and if that response is severe the tissue around it can be collateral damage.

A Leaky Brain Means More Brain Cells Get Chewed Up

The microglial cells also make up the blood-brain barrier, a thin barrier that lines the brain and only allows tiny, necessary substances to pass through.

The blood-brain barrier is important for keeping the bad guys (foreign invaders, such as viruses or bacteria) and environmental toxins out of the brain.

Unfortunately, according to Dr. Datis Kharrazian, (author of the book, *Why Isn't My Brain Working*) the blood-brain barrier can develop "leaks" for a variety of reasons.

These include poor blood-sugar stability (particularly insulin resistance), chronic stress, chronic inflammation, poor gut health, poor diet with unhealthy fats, and unchecked autoimmune activity, such as Hashimoto's disease (alcohol and high homocysteine are also recognized factors).

Brain Degeneration Can Also Be Autoimmune

Autoimmune attack on parts of the brain have also been noted with Hashimoto's patients.

One part of the brain that has been observed to be vulnerable in patients with Hashimoto's is the cerebellum. And as we have already seen, research has also shown that gluten can lead to destruction of the cerebellum (the Purkinje cells, in particular) through molecular mimicry (these cells resemble gluten proteins in structure).

Coincidence?

We have discussed the immune system in the brain above. Well, one thing that's important to understand is that it has no "off switch".

If there is an immune response in the brain there is nothing to call off the attack, and the microglial cells create brain inflammation and chew up brain tissue in the process.

What Does A Healthy Brain Need?

A healthy brain needs 3 things.

1. Oxygen
2. Glucose
3. Stimulation

1. Oxygen- In order to get sufficient amounts of oxygen to the brain you need to make sure you are getting sufficient blood flow to the brain. So things that inhibit blood flow can impact brain health.

Anemias, especially iron deficiency anemia, can lead to too little oxygen. If you are iron deficient, this must be corrected.

Low blood pressure can also reduce blood flow to the brain. If you're blood pressure is too low you may want to increase your salt consumption.

Smoking can also reduce blood flow to your brain.

You blood carries everything your brain needs: oxygen, glucose, nutrients, hormones and neurotransmitters.

Exercise is really important for improving brain health and circulation. High intensity for short duration may be most beneficial. About 5 minutes of high intensity per day is a good place to start.

2. Glucose- Up to 1/2 of the body's glucose supply fuels your brain.

If you are hypoglycemic and you go too long without eating, then you experience the effects of low glucose on the brain: feeling spacey, light headed, dull or slow-witted.

On the other hand, if you are a sugar addict and you have developed insulin resistance (the most common symptom of this is fatigue after meals) then glucose can't get into your cells and do it's job.

Either way, your brain suffers and brain cells get killed as a result.

So, if you are hypoglycemic, you must start the day with a good protein and fat combination and you must eat frequently throughout the day.

Your goal must be to never experience that spacey, light headed feeling again. By the time you experience that, it's too late. The damage has already been done.

For sugar addicts and those with hypoglycemia, a low carb diet like the Autoimmune Paleo approach is absolutely imperative.

3. Stimulation:

For stimulation, you need to do things that stimulate your brain in a variety of ways. Exercise is one way.

Games are another: Crossword puzzles, chess, memory games and other games that require mental activity are helpful. Web based brain games like **Lumosity.com** can various kinds of brain stimulation.

Hashimoto's and Brain Degeneration Are Both Multi-System Problems

One of the things that I frequently discuss in my writing and in my consultations is that Hashimoto's is a multi-system disorder.

It's not just a thyroid problem or just an immune system problem.

It extends into all the major systems of the body including the liver, the adrenals, the pancreas, the stomach, the digestive tract and, yes, the brain.

And this is often why people don't get better. Their doctors ignore all these other systems that are breaking down and just keep increasing the dosage of their thyroid hormone.

Well, a lot of times that just doesn't work. You need to have a multi-system strategy.

We really need a strategy for first determining where the problems are and then a program designed to fix them.

The A.P.A.R.T. System is designed to help you do this.

What Can You Do About Brain Degeneration?

You have to start by addressing the areas that helped cause a leaky blood-brain barrier if you want to restore brain integrity.

That's why we recommend the elimination phase of the Autoimmune Paleo Diet to determine whether other foods besides gluten, such as dairy or eggs, are also provoking the immune system.

Then we work on the other systems that are involved.

For example, balancing blood sugar, addressing gut health and gut infections, and supporting adrenal health so your adrenal hormones are neither too high or too low.

All of these will help put out the fires of inflammation, the killer of brain cells.

In addition, we use supplements created specifically for blood-brain barrier integrity for healing the leaky brain, brain inflammation for reducing inflammation in the brain and increased blood flow to the brain- the brain needs oxygen.

And we may also work on other strategies like enhancing the liver's methylation pathway and supplementing with alpha-lipoic acid.

And below you'll find some important questions to ask in order to properly evaluate the brain and brain nutrition.

The good news is, many of the things that we've discussed that are really beneficial for healing Hashimoto's are also really beneficial for the brain.

Now, let's dig deeper and see if there's anything else we need to do. Before we do that, let's do a quick recap.

Hashimoto's & the Brain Recap

1. A lot of common symptoms of Hashimoto's, like fatigue, brain fog and memory issues, poor concentration and emotional issues like depression, anxiety and moodiness, in general are all brain related (in the next part we're going to look more deeply at that stuff)

2. Some brain related issues have to do with hypothyroidism or functional hypothyroidism-not getting enough active thyroid hormone to brain cells.

3. Other brain related issues are related to autoimmunity in the brain. And gluten is a major player in this, as is dairy, by the way.

Dairy is very similar in protein structure to myeline, which is what surrounds nerves and neurons in the brain. If your immune system attacks dairy, it can attack the brain.

4. The brain needs 3 things to be healthy: oxygen, sugar and stimulation. Make sure you are not anemic, or have too low blood pressure. Also, be sure you balance your blood sugar and you get plenty of stimulation.

5. Lastly, all the things that make Hashimoto's worse, also make brain degeneration and inflammation of the brain worse. So we have to work on this.

Also, if you haven't seen it, make sure you check out my interview with Dr. Datis Kharrazian, author of a fantastic new book called Why Isn't My Brain Working? It's a great discussion about lots of these issues. You'll find that in the supplemental section on our website. Visit: https://hashimotos-diet.com/roadmap-to-remission-supplemental/

Ok, now we're going to take a look at some of the ways that Hashimoto's can impact the brain and how that can affect us emotionally and psychologically.

This is really important because a lot of people with this disease really struggle with feeling like they're crazy or they blame themselves for the way they feel and a lot of times, the reasons they feel this way are rooted in what's happening to our brains.

Chapter Nineteen

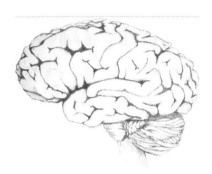

Neurotransmitters:
Molecules of Emotion

In this section, we're going to take a look at how all of this affects your emotions and your outlook.

In the other chapters, I also explore the Chinese medical perspective, but there isn't a whole lot related to the brain or the nervous system in Chinese medicine.

Traditionally, the brain is known as the sea of marrow or the sea of neural tissue.

In the Taoist tradition the glands in the brain have important spiritual meaning and power. Right? The pituitary and the hypothalmus- which we learned were so important for the adrenals and the thyroid are thought to be what is activated in meditation.

This area of the brain is thought to give and receive light and to awaken our inner knowledge. It here that we can get in touch with our deepest potentials.

So there was a sense from the Taoists of the mystical power of the brain. And I think we're really starting to see that with modern neuroscience.

I recently read a fascinating book called The Emotional Life of Your Brain by Richard Davidson. I highly recommend it.

He's a researcher and for 30 years he's done a lot of really interesting research on neuroscience and the brain. And, his research looks at the role of emotions in the brain.

And the first thing he writes in the book is that no two brains are alike and, therefore, no two people are alike.

I know this from clinical experience and if you've observed any of the Hashimoto's or thyroid support groups, you'll see this playing out every day.

Nothing works for everyone. No medication, no supplements, no diet is fool proof. And it all happens in degrees, right?

Sometimes they work perfectly, sometimes they work a little, sometimes they work great and then stop working, and sometimes they don't work at all.

You see this playing out over and over and over again. And one of the important reasons is the different ways that people's brains are wired.

One of the things the book makes clear is how complex this is. Like everything else, there are all these different things that affect the way you deal with things.

One of the most important, in dealing with Hashimoto's and the process of healing it, is how you deal with the challenges and the adversity of the disease.

Because, as it progresses, you will have plenty of opportunities for failure and disappointment.

I've worked with a lot of different people at different stages of Hashimoto's and what's interesting is some get results and some don't.

Or maybe a better way to say it is that some people with the same set of symptoms just get better results.

And as someone who has this disease himself and who has been through a good deal of adversity. I really want to help others avoid the same fate.

The thing this book really helped me to see is that the reason different people have different results is really dependent on the wiring of their brains.

Emotional Style: What's Yours?

There's this thing he calls Emotional Style and there are 6 different categories of things: how fast you recover, how resilient you are, what your outlook tends to be (are you generally positive or negative), how self-aware you are, how well you focus, etc..

And when you see this laid out, it all makes sense. This is a big part of why some people get better faster. It's not one thing.

Just like working on the physical part of Hashimoto's, there's all these different factors.

So first you have to figure out where you are in this spectrum, and that gives you a much better sense of where you need to go.

I just want you to think about that and realize that there are a number of different reasons why your brain wiring may be preventing you from getting the results that you want.

And, as you begin to figure out your emotional style, what's really unique to you, there are a few general truths that can be quite helpful.

And the first one has to do with learning.

Because one of the most important things that Hashimoto's has taught me is that I have to learn how to do things differently.

And real learning involves changing my behavior.

I can get some great advice about changes I need to make in my life, but if I don't change my behavior, I haven't learned anything. A perfect example of this is an alcoholic.

An alcoholic, hopefully, at some point knows he or she has to stop drinking. It becomes pretty obvious.

They have to have enough self-awareness to admit it, but eventually, if they do they know they have to change. And one of the best tools for changing the lives of alcoholics is Alcoholics Anonymous.

Because AA is a program that is entirely devoted to changing behavior. It's a system for real learning.

The ones that stay sober are those who learned how to live differently.

The same is true with Hashimoto's. You have to be able to learn and that means be able to change your behavior.

Around a lot of different things: food - things like gluten and sugar.

Thinking and language- the way you talk. That behavior often needs changing too.

How you speak to others and to yourself about your Hashimoto's can make a big difference.

How You Identify Yourself Matters

How do you identify yourself? Do you say things like "I'm a Hashi's." Well, stop for a second.

Are you really? If that's the case that means you are really strongly identifying yourself with the disease.

What can you say instead? I don't like using the word "Hashi's". To me, it's too cute. I don't want to get that close to it. It's always going to be Hashimoto's. I'd rather distance myself.

I have Hashimoto's. Or even better "I'm working on getting Hashimoto's in remission."

I often talk about that because that's my goal, that's my focus. In remission is somewhere over there, outside of me. That's where I want it.

Sometimes, I've observed people sometimes use all-or-nothing language: "I will never lose a pound, even if I live on celery!"

Or "I'm always tired, and nothing helps."

"I've tried everything, I've spent thousands of dollars. Nothing worked."

266

Talking like this wires your brain and reinforces these beliefs. It creates neural pathways that when reinforced often enough can create a positive feedback loop. This message can become self-fulfilling.

That becomes your default thought and what you keep saying. And if that becomes your default thought, then that becomes your reality.

Even if you're frustrated and you're not happy with where you are, you have to find a different way of expressing it.

"I'm not where I'd like to be yet." Something like that has a grain of hope.

Because it won't get better if you can't change your relationship to it. And I guarantee you, there is something that is better.

Something.

That's why a gratitude list can be a valuable habit to cultivate. Think about what you have to be grateful for and focus on it. That can dramatically change your relationship to this process.

The last thing I want to talk about is stress.

Stress and the Brain

We touched on this when we looked at the Water Element. And when we release too much cortisol as a result of being stressed, it can actually damage the brain and the body.

Hahsimoto's is at its root a disease of inflammation. And inflammatory markers like plasma fibrinogen rise during stressful events.

Stress is a major trigger of autoimmunity. And in terms of the brain, emotion plays a big role in impacting the immune system. Some neurons in the brain called sympathetic fibers, connect all the way to the thymus and lymph nodes.

So, activating these neurons in the brain with positive emotions like joy, happiness, enthusiasm, silliness, fun (is that an emotion?) has been shown to modulate the endocrine and immune systems.

That's our wheelhouse. Hashimoto's is an autoimmune disease of the endocrine gland.

How your brain is wired can have a big impact on healing. And what's really interesting is that with the mind-body connection it's not just a one way thing.

What happens in your brain affects your body and what happens in your body affects your brain. So everything you're learning, it's not just woo woo or theoretical, it's grounded in science.

Ok, the second area I wanted to look at is how hypothyroidism and Hashimoto's can lead to deficiencies in important neurotransmitters.

Molecules of Emotion

Well, these are the "molecules of emotion" as researcher and scientist Candace Pert, discoverer of the opiate receptor in the brain, called them in her book of the same name, Molecules of Emotion.

Why should you care about all of this?

Because as we learn about your emotional style, we can discover whether you're resilient, hopeful or focused. Deficiencies in any of these neurotransmitters can affect these emotions and behaviors.

If you have these deficiencies, then your odds of improving your thinking or your behavior are greatly reduced.

If you want to succeed, you have to work to make the odds in your favor. Right?

I don't know about you, but I'd rather go to the track knowing which horse has the advantage.

I like to win, its more fun.

So if you want to be more resilient and have a better outlook, or be more focused you should make sure you enough of the neurotransmitters that make these things happen.

There are many, but the ones that we're going to look at are serotonin, dopamine, acetylcholine, and GABA.

What Is a Neurotransmitter?

A neurotransmitter is a compound released from a nerve terminal.

When an electrical impulse travels to the end of a nerve cell, it stimulates the terminal of this cell to secrete a chemical signaling molecule at a special place between nerve cells called a synapse.

What happens with these signaling chemicals is they make us feel stuff. And with hypothyroidism, we can easily become deficient in them.

This is what makes your emotions go all over the map. As we have seen, depression and anxiety are very common with Hashimoto's patients.

The reason these people are feeling this way is because of this connection between thyroid hormone and these neurotransmitters.

Serotonin

Too little serotonin can make you feel sadness, rage, loss of enjoyment in things, you may just feel like giving up. It makes you less resilient.

Serotonin is also used as a messenger to release TSH, and it modulates the production of T3 inside cells using an enzyme called 5' deodinase. It actually may influence the rate of T3 conversion.

And it works the other way too. Thyroid hormone has a direct effect on the amount of serotonin is your body and if you have too little thyroid hormone, this slows the synthesis of serotonin.

This is one reason that some people with hypothyroidism and functional hypothyroidism get depressed.

There's always a physiological reason, people. It's not becasue you're just depressed.

This depression can be caused by too little serotonin.

And a lot of anti-depressants work by blocking the re-uptake of serotonin. It floods your body with more of it.

Dopamine

Too little dopamine can make you feel self destructive thoughts, isolation, anger and irritability. It's the reward and pleasure molecule.

Drug addiction is the same thing as being a dopamine fiend.

Too little dopamine makes you feel like, why bother? There's no reward. With serotonin deficiency you just can't find joy. With dopamine deficiency you can get joy, but you just feel like, What's the point?

Thyroid hormones play an important role in the release of dopamine. And studies have shown that reduced dopamine can actually raise TSH. This is yet another reason why this test is sometimes not reliable for checking on how your thyroid is doing.

Your thyroid doesn't exist in a vacuum. Its interacting with all these other things: neurotransmitters, other endocrine glands like the adrenals and the pituitary and the pancreas. And the brain.

Acetylcholine

This is a really important neurotransmitter for brain activity. It's responsible for nerve firing.

Too little acetylcholine can cause memory issues, slow recall, difficulty calculating, and problems with focus. Having trouble paying attention right now?

Could be you are deficient in acetylcholine.

When you are hypothyroid, your brain uses acetylcholine to make up for insufficient amounts of thyroid hormone. It's like borrowing from Peter to pay Paul.

T3 has been found to directly stimulate acetylcholine.

This is one of those neurotransmitters that I take supplements for on a regular basis. It's great for ADD or ADHD.

GABA

GABA stands for gamma-aminobutryic acid.

And too little GABA can make you feel anxiety, panic, and restlessness.

It's calming. Therefore, too little makes you uptight and not in a good way.

It also affects TSH release in the pituitary. It affects how much TSH is released. It also affects thyroid hormones that are stimulated by TSH.
Like T4.

And thyroid hormones keep GABA in your system after it is released and make more of it get released.

Again, this all goes both ways.

You're Not Crazy!

You're not crazy, it's the impact of hypothyroidism on your brain and these neurotransmitters.

If you have too little serotonin that will impact your ability to bounce back and whether or not you get enjoyment and pleasure from things.

Too little dopamine is going to impact your outlook and your motivation.

Too little acetylcholine means you can't focus or concentrate and finish tasks. Making changes requires focus.

Too little GABA will make you unable to handle stressors. You may freak out on a regular basis over trivial things. This can lead to anxiety or worry.

We have to look for these things. Not pretend this isn't happening. It's happening, all the time.

All of these neurotransmitters can be nourished. You can take the raw materials for them to help your body produce more of them when you're deficient.

(I've put a list of some of the food sources of the building blocks of these neurotransmitters in the final chapter of this section.)

This is way more than a thyroid problem. It's an all over your body problem and that's where the answers are.

You see? It is all connected, all the physical issues, all the emotional issues, the way you feel.

It's all happening for a reason and that reason is the impact that this is having on our minds, our bodies and our spirits.

So take a moment and forgive yourself. It's not your fault.

Chapter Twenty

Using the A.P.A.R.T. System to Save Your Brain

The A.P.A.R.T. System

1. A = Ask and Asses

Grab your journal and look for symptoms of problems with the brain. Note what they are, then create a plan for addressing them. After that, you must act on your plan. Follow through and do what you have planned.

After that take inventory of what you did. Look at what worked and what didn't. Both will provide valuable information.

Double down on what worked, change what didn't. Don't ever stop this process. Your brain is too important.

Brain Related Symptoms

Low Circulation: Low blood pressure, Low brain endurance for focus and concentration, Cold hands and feet, Poor nail health, Fungal growth on toenails, Must wear socks at night, The tip of the nose is cold

Essential Fatty Acid Deficiency: Dry and unhealthy skin, Dandruff or a flaky scalp, Consumption of processed foods that are bagged or boxed, Consumption of fried foods, Difficulty consuming raw nuts or seeds, Difficulty consuming fish (not fried).

Also if you have Gall Bladder Issues you may have difficulty consuming olive oil, avocados, flax seed oil, or natural fats (this can lead to deficiencies in these natural fats)

Hypoglycemia Irritable, nervous, shaky, or light headed between meals, Feel energized after meals, Difficulty eating large meals in the morning ,Energy level drops in the afternoon, Crave sugar and sweets in the afternoon, Wake up in the middle of the night, Difficulty concentrating before eating, Depend on coffee and sugar for energy

Insulin resistance: Fatigue after meals, Sugar and sweet cravings after meals, Need for stimulant, such as coffee, after meals, difficulty losing weight, Increased frequency of urination, Difficulty losing weight, Difficulty falling asleep, Increased appetite

Neurotransmitter Symptoms:

The best way to assess neurotransmitters is to look at the symptoms associated with them. There is saliva testing available for neurotransmitters but the science on it is questionable.

Instead, get out your journal, and write down the symptoms that you have. Determine which might be deficient and try some of the recommendations below.

Serotonin: Key symptoms include: A loss of pleasure in hobbies and interests, Feeling overwhelmed with ideas to manage, Feelings of inner rage or unprovoked anger, paranoia, sadness for no reason, A loss of enjoyment in various things like favorite activities, favorite foods, friendships and relationships, Feelings of susceptibility to pain

Dopamine: Key symptoms include: A feeling like "What's the point? There's nothing in it for me", Feelings of worthlessness, and hopelessness, Self destructive thoughts, Inability to handle stress, Or getting angry and aggressive when stressed, A desire to isolate yourself from others, An unexplained lack of concern for family and friends, An inability to finish tasks, Feelings of anger for minor reasons

Acetylecholine: Key symptoms include: Memory issues (especially short term), A decrease in visual memory (shapes and images) and verbal memory, Occurrence of memory lapses, Difficulty calculating numbers, Difficulty recognizing objects and faces, Slow mental recall

Catecholamines: Key symptoms include: Needing coffee or caffeine sources to improve mental function A decrease in mental alertness, and speed, A decrease in concentration quality, Slow cognitive processing, An increase in the ability to be distracted

GABA: Key symptoms include: Feelings of nervousness or panic for no reason, Feelings of dread, Feelings of a "knot" in your stomach, Feelings of being overwhelmed for no reason, An inability to turn off the mind when relaxing, Disorganized attention, Worry over things never thought about before, Feelings of inner tension and inner excitability

2. P = Prioritize and Plan

Not everything has the same level importance. This is what 80/20 teaches us. Some things are having more of an impact than others. Figure out which they are (the positive feedback loops) and then make a plan to fix them.

There is an awful lot to unpack when it comes to the brain. There's inflammation, autoimmunity, neurotransmitters, possible permeability to the blood brain barrier.

All of these things need to be evaluated and treated. Without question, this is a top priority.

3. A = Act and Adapt

Act and put your plan into motion. Then observe what the results are.

First step? The Autoimmune Paleo Diet.

Why is the Autoimmune Paleo Diet a good diet for the brain?

So glad you asked. :) It helps address the major needs of a healthy brain.

The brain needs 3 things:

1. Oxygen
2. Glucose
3. Healthy Amounts of Blood

1. Oxygen: In order to get oxygen to the brain you must have healthy blood pressure and good blood flow.

If you haven't done so, check your blood pressure. Normal range is 120/80. If you are 10 points or lower than that, then you may need to do something to raise your blood pressure.

A little sea salt or Himalayan salt can be helpful.

Check below for other important recommendations on this.

2. Sugar: Sugar is a huge issue for the brain. And this can be a problem both if you have too much or too little.

So, if you are hypoglycemic, you cannot skip meals or go long periods without eating. When you do this, you deprive your brain of important fuel.

That spacey, irritable, feeling is your brain saying, "What are you doing to me?" That can cause brain inflammation, which by now, I hope you realize is not good.

The flip side of this is too much sugar or insulin resistance. While your brain definitely needs sugar, too much sugar is brain poison.

It is also inflammatory and if you routinely take in too much sugar, you may develop insulin resistance which means insulin can't get into your cells, which means sugar can't get in and do it's job either.

And, researchers now believe that excess sugar is a major causative factor in Alzheimer's. In fact, they are actually calling it Brain Diabetes or Type III Diabetes.

In a review of the literature published in the Journal of Diabetes Science and Technology November 2008, Susan M. Dela Monte MD and Jack R Wands MD concluded: "Altogether, the results from these studies provide strong evidence in support of the hypothesis that AD (Alzheimer's Disease) represents a form of diabetes mellitus that selectively afflicts the brain."

It's no joke. You have to take sugar seriously. We've seen how it can make Hashimoto's so much worse. Well, if that's not incentive enough, it can also destroy your brain.

And the Autoimmune Paleo diet can really help correct this. It takes all refined sugar out of your diet and helps to convert you from a sugar burner to a fat burner.

3. Oxygen: The last point is also hugely important for the brain. The brain needs blood flow. And if you are anemic, iron deficient of B12 or B6 deficient this compromises your brain.

You don't get essential nutrients and you don't get enough red blood cells (Which carry oxygen) to your brain.

YOU CANNOT BE ANEMIC AT ALL!

Not even a little. Seriously, this is super important.

Foods for the Brain and Neurotransmitters:

Dietary Sources of DHA & EPA

EPA- Fish, fish oils, Marine sources

279

DHA- Fish, Fish oils, Specialty egg/dairy products

Fish- Anchovy, Carp, Catfish, Cod, Eel, Flatfish, Haddock, Halibut, Herring, Mackerel, Mullet, Perch, Pike, Pollock, Salmon, Sardine, Sea bass, Shark, Snapper, Swordfish, Trout, Tuna, Whiting

Crustaceans- Crab, Shrimp, Spiny lobster

Mollusks- Clam, Conch, Mussel, Octopus, Oyster, Scallop

Be cautious with Fish, make sure to have variety and to eat more smaller fish which are lower on the food chain and less likely to have accumulated heavy metals and other environmental toxins.

Serotonin

Foods that are high in the amino acid tryptophan (a precursor for serotonin):

Avocado, Wild game, Chicken, Duck, Pork, Turkey

Vitamins and Supplements for Serotonoin:

Calcium, Fish oils, 5-HTP, Magnesium, Melatonin, Passionflower, Pyridoxine, SAM-e, St. John's wort, Tryptophan, Zinc

Avoid: PCBs, pesticides and rinse all produce thoroughly, preferably eat grass fed, organic meat.

Dopamine:

Meat: chicken, duck, turkey

(Do not eat these foods when doing the elimination phase of the diet): Dark chocolate, walnuts, eggs

Vitamins and Supplements Dopamine:

Phenylalanine, Tyrosine, Methionine, Rhodiola, Pyridoxine, B complex, Phosphatidylserine, Ginkgo biloba

Rhodiola is an adaptogen. It can enhance concentration and endurance, uplifting one's mental state and supporting optimal immune, adrenal cardiovascular function even under conditions of severe stress.

Avoid: Avoid cigarette smoke and quit smoking as cadmium in cigarettes reduces dopamine

Acetylcholine:

Avocado, Artichokes, Beef, Broccoli, Brussels sprouts, Cabbage, Cucumber, Eggs, Fish, Liver, Lettuce, Zucchini

Supplements:

These are best taken early in the morning through the afternoon.

Choline, Phosphatidylcholine, Phosphatidylserine, Acetyl –L-carnitine, DHA, Thiamine, Pantothenic acid, Vitamin B12, Taurine, Huperzine-A, Ginkgo bilboba, Korean ginseng

Avoid: aluminum, fluorescent lighting and change to full spectrum lights, avoid or shield yourself from EMF's from computers, cell phones, power lines, microwaves

GABA

Foods high in glutamic acid/glutamate:

Banana, Beef liver, Broccoli, Spinach, Oranges, Halibut

People with GABA issues should avoid simple carbohydrates such as simple sugars, white flour and wheat products.

GABA Vitamins and Supplements:

Inositol, GABA, Glutamic acid, Thiamine, Niacinamide, Pyridoxine, Valerian root, Passionflower

Avoid: lead and toxic chemicals

Exercises for the Brain

Simple Qi Gong exercise for the brain:

Beating the Heavenly Drum – Place palm over ears with finger spread over back of head. Overlap and snap the index and middle fingers over each other and gently hit the back of your skull with your index finger. 9 times. This exercise stimulates the brain, prevents stroke, and improves memory.

Exercise Tips for Neurotransmitters:

Serotonin: Aerobic exercise, prayer, meditation, yoga, chanting

Dopamine: Weight lifting, meditation and relaxation, alternate nostril breathing

Acetylcholine: Aerobic exercise, Soft lighting, gentle music, pleasant scents

GABA: Aerobic exercise, play and recreation, allow others to take care of you

4. R= Reassess and Readjust

Retest, Reassess and ask all over again. Figure out what worked and what didn't. Double down on what worked and either eliminate or recreate a plan for what didn't.

Since there are no reliable laboratory tests for neurotransmitters, the best way to asses them is by looking at the symptoms associated with them.

Use your journal to get an initial assessment. Then try some of the things suggested and ask about those symptoms again.

5. T = Try and Try Again

Keep doing it, keep refining, keep building on the positive results and keep looking for the remaining positive feedback loops that are causing vicious cycles.

Chapter Twenty-One

The Wood Element:
Liver & Gall Bladder

In this chapter we'll be looking at the Wood Element which is the liver and gall bladder in Chinese medicine.

You'll discover how the thyroid and liver are so dependent on one another.

You'll learn what hormone medication can torpedo thyroid health. And how important healthy liver function is for clearing out these hormones.

You'll discover how to detoxify your liver and gall bladder in a gentle way so that they can effectively clear hormones, environmental toxins and pathogens that can make your symptoms worse.

The Yin and Yang of the Wood Element

The yin organ is the liver and the yang organ is the gall bladder. It's not hard to see how these 2 are related. They live together just underneath your ribcage on the right side of your torso.

Let's start with the liver. What an amazing organ this is!

Our Amazing Liver

In Chinese medicine, the liver was traditionally regarded as "the general" of the body because of its role in orchestrating so many important activities.

In fact, the liver is probably the most diverse and active organ in the body.

It performs many important functions and is the location where most of the major biochemical pathways used for both anabolic (building) or catabolic (breaking down) activity takes place.

The liver also functions as a filter to remove toxins and waste products from the body and it stores nutrients such as vitamins, minerals, and iron.

In addition, it plays a role in managing levels of certain chemicals in the body, such as cholesterol, hormones and sugars. A healthy liver filters about 1.5 quarts of blood per minute.

The liver is also centrally involved with carbohydrate, fat and protein metabolism. The liver's role in carbohydrate metabolism is to help the body maintain adequate levels of sugar.

The liver's role in fat metabolism involves a number of important reactions. First, the liver is very active in oxidizing triglycerides (sugars stored as fat) to produce energy.

The liver is also responsible for the bulk of lipoprotein production and lipogenesis (the process by which simple sugars such as glucose are converted to fatty acids) when the body has to convert excess glucose and proteins into fat. The liver also synthesizes large quantities of cholesterol and phospholipids.

> *It is interesting to note that low fat diets and products that have been heavily marketed for years do not actually address the real problem, sugar.*

Fat in the Liver Is Caused By Too Much Sugar

The reason why we have so many problems regarding fat accumulation in the liver (fatty liver) is because of the excessive amounts of sugar in the typical American diet.

Even many "low fat" foods have lots of sugar added to them, most of which is often in the form of high fructose corn syrup that is almost entirely converted into fat in the liver.

Hopefully, you've already gotten a sense of how destructive sugar imbalances can be for people with Hashimoto's. But if you needed extra incentive to get off of sugar, it's also the major cause of fatty liver disease and elevated fats like triglycerides, cholesterol and LDL.

CASE STUDY: HOW IMPROVING LIVER FUNCTION CAN HELP LOWER CHOLESTEROL

Patient is a 57 year old female with Hashimoto's who presented with high cholesterol, high LDL and triglycerides. (Used with permission)

Her main concerns were weight gain, difficulty sleeping, shortness of breath, and upper back pain.

She was also experiencing constipation and sluggish bowels, exhaustion in the morning (in fact she sometimes feels like she didn't get any sleep even when she has). She also would get winded and tired very easily. Walking up hill would wipe her out sometimes.

She was prescribed Armour thyroid and all her thyroid numbers were in the normal range. In the past she had tried Synthroid and did not react well to it.

After a workup of all the systems of her body, we elected to focus on healing the gut, nourishing detoxification pathways in the liver, reducing systemic inflammation and on healing her adrenals.

The goal was to improve function in these areas and then to revisit the cholesterol after we had done this.

About 60 days later she got another blood test and her cholesterol had dropped over 100 points (it went from 320 to 218).

What did we do?

Got her on a strict Autoimmune Paleo diet which effectively eliminated all the refined sugars that were driving her high cholesterol.

We improved liver function and reduced systemic inflammation, thereby helping her thyroid medication work better.

And we worked on healing her adrenals so she had some energy.

Liver and Protein Metabolism

Finally, the liver is involved in some important aspects of protein metabolism. First, it is active in the breakdown of amino acids and it is because of this that liver "transaminase" enzymes such as ALT are measured to assess liver disease.

Liver cells are also responsible for the synthesis of plasma proteins such as albumin. Albumin and clotting factor are only made in the liver, so tests measuring serum albumin and prothombin time are also excellent for assessing liver function and health.

In addition, the liver plays an important role in the removal of waste products of protein such as ammonia. When the liver fails to function properly, the body fills with excess amounts of ammonia, which can lead to impaired brain function due to advanced liver damage.

The liver is also very important in dealing with environmental toxins. In the medical literature this is known as biotransformation, most other folks call it detoxification or detox. We'll get deeper into this in a moment.

Liver and Hashimoto's

As always we must ask, how does this relate to Hashimoto's?

The body is not a machine, like our earth it is a group of interacting ecosystems that all talk to one another and influence each other in both good and bad ways.

289

The liver and the thyroid are a perfect example of this. Here is a brief breakdown of how they interact:

---

* 60% of thyroid hormone is converted from T4 to T3 in the liver. Both T3 and T4 are glucoronidated and sulfated there. (More on that in a minute).

* Thyroid hormone influences the way that cholesterol and other lipids are synthesized and broken down (and where does this happen? – yes, the liver).

With Hashimoto's and hypothyroidism, this is often slowed down resulting in high cholesterol and other lipids like LDL and triglycerides.

* Thyroid hormone affects detoxification pathways in the liver and affects insulin growth factor and cytochrome P450 enzymes which metabolize lots of drugs and environmental toxins. When this slows you can have toxins build up.

* On the autoimmune side, Huang et al have noted in the Journal of Gastroenterology and Hepatology that there is a link between autoimmune thyroid and autoimmune liver diseases, and that the liver and the thyroid are mutually responsible for proper function in each other.

*Very high levels of thyroid hormone (T3) can raise bilirubin levels and can actually be toxic to the liver because it damages mitochondria.

How Is Thyroid Hormone Converted in the Liver?

Thyroid hormones are converted into their usable form in the liver (60% happens there), you can see how low thyroid function can create a vicious cycle.

Hypothyroidism impairs liver function and fewer thyroid hormones become active. So it goes until you have all of the common symptoms of too little thyroid hormone: fatigue, brain fog, joint pain, hair loss, weight gain, depression, etc.

290

Thyroid hormone is converted primarily through 2 processes: Glucornidation and sulfation, let's break these down.

Glucoronidation

Glucoronidation is an important process for converting thyroid hormone. This pathway is supported by B vitamins, magnesium, and glassine.

Sulfation

Sulfation involves binding things partially broken down in the liver with sulfur containing compounds. It is one of the major detoxification pathways for neurotransmitters, toxins, and hormones (like thyroid hormones).

Vitamin B6 and magnesium are important for sulfur amino acid metabolism, as are foods containing sulfur such as: eggs, meat, poultry, nuts and legumes.

Its important to choose animals products wisely, buy organic whenever possible because organic foods have far fewer toxins like antibiotics, hormones, and pesticides which can all cause problems with the liver.

Another important point about sulfating is that it requires sulfate which is often poorly absorbed by the digestive system, especially by people with Hashimoto's who often suffer from leaky gut syndrome.

Sulfate is the oxidized, inorganic form of sulfur produced by an oxidation step called (you guessed it) sulfoxidation.

This step is made possible by an enzyme that is called sulfite oxidase which uses the essential mineral molybdenum. Problems with sulfoxidation can be seen in people who are sensitive to foods that contain sulfites (garlic) or drugs and food additives (in dried fruit and herbs, preservatives, in salad bars used to keep vegetables looking fresh).

(These people may also have an abnormally strong odor in their urine after eating asparagus. For these people one should consider molybdenum supplementation or organic sulfates like sodium sulfate or magnesium sulfate.)

The liver is such a valuable organ and it takes such a beating in today's world. So many things give it a hard time.

Chemicals, heavy metals, drugs, food additives, jeez, poor thing. I love you liver! (I'm just going to come out and say it. I don't care who knows.)

Recap: What the Liver Does

1. The liver is like the general of the body. It is involved in orchestrating protein, carbohydrate and fat storage and production.

2. It is heavily involved in biotransformation or detoxification and, Lord knows, we need to know how to detox our poor livers.

3. The liver does all kinds of stuff related to the thyroid: It is where most of the conversion of T4 to T3 happens (60%).

4. And thyroid hormone has a big impact on activities in the liver: it affects cholesterol production and metabolism, it affects detoxification and too much T3 can actually be toxic to the liver.

5. Thyroid hormone is converted via 2 main pathways: glucoronidation and sulfation.

Love your liver. Be a liver lover. Love you liver!

Chapter Twenty-Two

The Gall Bladder & Liver Detoxification

Let's take a look at the gallbladder in all of this: The gallbladder is a small pear shaped sac located just below the liver and it stores and concentrates bile. It is connected to the liver (which produces the bile) by the hepatic duct.

When food that contains fat reaches the small intestine, a hormone is produced by cells in the intestinal wall and carried to the gall bladder via the bloodstream.

The hormone (cholecystokin-for you curious readers) causes the gallbladder to contract, forcing bile into the common bile duct.

A valve, which opens only when food is present in the intestine, allows bile to flow from the common bile duct to the duodenum (located in the upper small intestine) where it functions in the process of fat digestion.

Sometimes substances contained in bile crystallize in the gallbladder and this forms gall stones. These small hard objects are more common in persons over 40, especially in women and the obese.

These stones can cause inflammation in the gallbladder, a disorder that produces symptoms similar to indigestion, and these are often worse after a fatty meal.

How Does the Gall Bladder Fit In to This?

The liver has several pathways through which it metabolizes hormones, filters toxins, and cleans the blood. Byproducts from these processes are dumped into the gall bladder to help get them out of the body.

Low thyroid function slows down this whole process, making the liver and gall bladder sluggish and congested and helping to make gallstones.

Gallbladder x-rays in hypothyroid patients can show a bloated gall bladder that contracts sluggishly.

This can slow down the flow of bile which can lead to slower breakdown of fats and cholesterol and other toxins that are broken down in the liver.

This whole process can also lead to the formation of gall stones. Many people with Hashimoto's have gall bladder issues.

Another important area for Hashimoto's folks is liver detoxification. If liver detoxification is not addressed treatment will often not work or success will be severely limited.

For example, as many of us know, much of conventional healthcare treatment looks at lab test results to determine which hormones a person is deficient in.

With Hashimoto's, as we've seen, its usually TSH and sometimes T4, if you're lucky.

Most therapy is aimed at giving the same hormone therapies to everyone. As we have also seen, it's usually synthetic T4. The truth is, however, that many hormonal imbalances are there because of compromised detoxification function.

This is especially true when a patient's blood work does not match their symptoms or if they have a previous history of toxic overload in the form of chemical or drug exposure.

> **In addition, if people have detoxification issues that are causing their problems, using hormones or drugs may make their problems worse.**

Unfortunately, a very common approach used by many physicians ignores these detoxification issues and they just continue to increase the dosage of thyroid hormone.

Well, if your liver is not functioning properly this can result in more adverse reactions like increased hair loss, increase loss of bone density, palpitations, irregular heart beat, insomnia, anxiety and much more.

And this is not limited to hormonal issues, this may be true for many different health problems.

For example, many studies have shown that poor detoxification can lead to neurological disorders, chemical sensitivities, adverse drug reactions, fatigue, and auto-immune disorders.

If proper liver detoxification is not restored, the chances of returning a person back to optimal health are really low. This is not to say that this is a simple process, there are many factors involved.

Liver Detoxification

Liver Detoxification involves 2 basic steps called Phase I and Phase II. There is also what could be termed Phase III and this involves the gallbladder.

Phase I Detoxification
The ultimate goal of detoxification in the liver is to take fat soluble compounds and change them into water soluble compounds and the use bile so that they can be excreted by the kidneys in the urine, in sweat, and through

the bowels as feces.

These compounds (called lipophilic chemicals - meaning fat loving - love me some fat!) come from sources inside the body, such as: hormones, neurotransmitters, stuff inside cells (calcium, sodium, potassium, etc.), also from bacteria, toxins produced by intestinal bacteria, and broken down immune complexes (like antibodies and antigens).

The liver also transforms chemicals from outside the body like drugs, pesticides, and environmental toxins, etc. into these same water soluble compounds so that they can be eliminated from the body.

Phase I detoxification involves enzymes called cytochrome 450 enzymes. They directly neutralize some chemicals, but most others are changed into these intermediate forms that are then converted by what are called phase II enzymes.

This process is what is called "conjugation". It is interesting to note that once a compound has been converted by a phase I enzyme into this in-between form, it becomes much more active and toxic.

OK? Stay with me.

So, some people have very active phase I detoxification systems and slow or inactive phase II enzymes.

These are the people who may have severe reactions to toxins and they often suffer some chronic pain or illness. One side effect of phase I deactivation of toxic compounds is free radical production.

For every molecule of toxin metabolized by phase I, one molecule of free radical is generated. This is why taking anti-oxidants are so important. They neutralize these free radicals.

One of the most important anti-oxidants is ....wait for it...glutathione; which we have already sung the praises of.

It is extremely important in neutralizing phase I side effects, and serving as a platform for phase II conjugation. The stuff is incredible.

Phase II Detoxification

Phase II liver detoxification usually involves the conjugation of these phase I half detoxed things, but some toxins are directly acted upon by phase II

298

enzymes.

This conjugation reaction either neutralizes the toxin or makes it more easily eliminated through the urine, bile or sweat.

There are 6 main phase II pathways including: glutathione conjugation, glycine conjugation, methylation, sulfation, acetylation and glucuronidation.

We've already looked at 2 of them, glucoronidation and sulfating because those are the pathways that convert thyroid hormone.

You see how this all connected?

For more information on these other pathways, visit the supplemental section on our website at https://hashimotos-diet.com/roadmap-to-remission-supplemental/

Phase III Detoxification

This involves the gall bladder. Once the liver has detoxified chemicals, they are delivered to the bile for elimination via the feces.

If there are problems with bile synthesis or secretion, liver detoxification of toxins, nasty chemicals and hormones will not be eliminated.

Improving bile function should be considered with anyone who complains of gallstone-type symptoms such as problems digesting fried foods, flatulence several hours after meals, excessive burping after meals, etc.

This should also be considered in people who have had their gall bladders removed. When this organ is removed, the cystic duct acts as a reservoir for bile.

Therefore, it is very important to have proper elimination of bile.

I get this question a lot. People often ask me. "Hey if I had my gall bladder removed do I still need to worry about this?"

Here's the thing: Just because a surgeon decided to remove an organ from your body does not mean that millions of years of evolution are magically made to disappear.

Your body still continues to function and still continues to need the services performed by that now missing body part.

Some other part of your body must compensate for this. In the case of your gall bladder, a portion of the duct is usually left and the liver adapts and takes up the functions previously done by the gall bladder.

Another interesting thing to note is that the body reabsorbs approximately 96% of the bile we produce. If this bile is still full of toxins you can continually recycle toxic bile.

Bile is made primarily of lecithin. So to build bile, eat more lecithin if you can tolerate it.

Bile Synthesis Helps Clear Hormones from the Body

And one last thing, bile synthesis and elimination can be very helpful when balancing hormones, due to its ability to help clear hormones out of the body.

And that brings me to one heck of a segue.

I want to talk about some medications that can really adversely affect thyroid function. The first being birth control, which can stay in the body for a prolonged period and just keep circulating. When this happens you can accumulate excess amount of estrogen that can cause problems with thyroid hormone absorption.

A year or so ago, I interviewed Dr. Izabella Wentz and we talked about her Book, Hashimoto's Thyroditis: Lifestyle Interventions for Finding and Treating the Root Cause. And one thing that came up was birth control.

Birth Control and Hashimoto's

Here's some information on this that I learned from her which comes from her book. Birth control pills can have big impact on thyroid and immune health and can be a major trigger for Hashimoto's.

They deplete the body of important nutrients that are essential for thyroid function like zinc, selenium and the amino acid tyrosine. In addition, they deplete the body of folic acid, vitamin B12, and B6.

Depletions of these vitamins can lead to anemias, depression and can impact how thyroid hormone is metabolized in the liver because these vitamins are necessary for conversion of T4 to T3.

Many oral contraceptives also contain lactose as an inactive filler. This may be a problem for women with Hashimoto's because many have dairy intolerances and this can cause a flare up of symptoms.

In addition, birth control pills can impact intestinal bacteria, allowing yeast and disruptive species to take over.

As we have seen, healthy intestinal bacteria is essential for proper thyroid hormone conversion and disruptions in the ecosystems of your gut can lead to additional immune dysfunction.

And finally, oral contraceptives actually simulate a shift from TH1 to TH2 because they create a state that is similar to pregnancy in the body. This can create more instability and confusion in the immune system.

And that's just 1 drug and that's only part of the impact it has on the body. These are the unintended consequences of medication.

Clinical Pearl: The best laboratory test for determining the impact of synthetic hormones and other synthetic drugs that can impact the thyroid is resin T3 Uptake.

This test measures the amount of receptor sites available for unbound T3 to bind on. This is critical for thyroid hormone to do its job. If there aren't enough of these sites available, thyroid hormone may not work properly.

This may be high or low: High T3 Uptake may be caused by heparin, anabolic steroids (testosterone), phentytoin, and large doses of salicylates (aspirin). High T3 uptake is found in hyperthyroidism.

Low T3 Uptake may be caused by normal pregnancy, heparin, estrogen, methadone and anti-ovulatory drugs. Low T3 Uptake is found in hypothyroidism.

There are other drugs that may reduce TSH secretion, decrease thyroid hormone secretions, and decrease T4 absorption: for example antacids. When you take antacids with levothyroxine with calcium carbonate it may form an insoluble new thing.

This means it can't be absorbed. We already discussed how common issues with acid reflux are with people with Hashimoto's. It is common for people to take antacids.

The same is true with ferris sulfate, an iron supplement, it may also hamper thyroid hormone absorption.

Other drugs like phenobarbital actually increase the liver's degradation of levothyroxine which means you may need a higher dosage to get the same result.

Metformin, a popular drug used for diabetes has been found to cross the blood brain barrier and impact the pituitary gland. It may suppress pituitary TSH in hypothyroid patients to subnormal levels.

And this is by no means a complete list.

In conclusion, we have two important things to think about With regard to medication and the liver. Firstly, a clogged liver may have difficulty in metabolizing and detoxifying hormones and medication which means you may have more of it circulating in your body or you may have more toxic metabolites that can intensify inflammation.

Secondly, you must always consider the effect of other medication that you have been prescribed on thyroid hormone. An excellent website for researching drug/drug interactions is rxlist.com.

Wow, we've covered a lot of information. Ok, let's recap.

Recap

1. Gall bladder function can be compromised with Hashimoto's. If you've had your gall bladder removed, the remaining duct and yhe liver must do the work of the old gall bladder.

In either case, supplements that help with bile flow (I've listed them in the supplemental materials) can really help.

2. Liver Detox: it's huge.

Phase I: Changes fat soluble substances into potent "in-between" super toxins that wait to be further transformed into water soluble substances so that your body can say, "Buh bye"

These "in-between" metabolites can cause real damage. Antioxidants help. Our buddy, glutathione, is the champ among champs in this regard.

Phase II: 6 different pathways to neutralize those scary in-between toxins or to just plain get them outta here!

Phase III: Bile gets in on the action. If you have a compromised gall bladder or a surgeon has decided to remove yours then eliminating toxins may not happen as well as it should. And you could be recycling these toxins.

Taking herbs and other things that help with bile flow may be a really good idea for these folks.

Lastly, many problems with drugs and hormones are caused by poor detoxification. If they can't be metabolized or eliminated properly they can stay in circulation and continue to be biologically and chemically active.

So, let's work on it people! Give those livers and gall bladders some love. Be a liver lover.

HASHIMOMENT:
DON'T STOP LOVING

Sometimes, with Hashimoto's we get frustrated and angry. Both at ourselves and others. It's a natural response to being out of control.

And Hashimoto's has a profound impact on our brains and on neurotransmitters, the molecules of emotion in our bodies.

This can make us moody, short tempered and inclined to lash out.
Or the fatigue, brain fog and the pain can make us not want to hang out and socialize because it's just too much effort.

But when you hurt others or yourself, you create another type of vicious cycle.

And this vicious cycle can be hard to break.

It feeds on itself.

One simple way to break it is to be kind and loving in spite of it all.

Don't forget to be compassionate to everyone, including yourself.

Chapter Twenty-Three

The Chinese Medicine View of the Wood Element

Now let's take a look at the wood element in the context of Chinese medicine. The liver is the yin organ and the gall bladder is the yang organ.

Sphere of Influence of the Liver

The nervous system, tendons and ligaments and the eyes are thought to be part of the sphere of influence of the liver.

And so many people with Hashimoto's also have issues in all of these areas: eye problems, tendon issues, and cognitive issues affecting the brain.

Most people associate eye issues with Grave's disease, but they are also a big problem for people with Hashimoto's. Severe eye pain was what first led me to my diagnosis.

Carpal tunnel syndrome is the most common tendon related issue connected to Hashimoto's. Often times getting off of gluten, dairy and soy can dramatically improve symptoms.

And, of course, brain issues are huge problem for people with Hashimoto's. As we have already seen, the familiar brain fog is often a sign of inflammation of the brain, but some people develop serious complications and brain degeneration from a condition called Hashimoto's Encephalitis.

As you know, in Chinese medicine, we view interactions in the body in the context of body, mind and spirit.

This can be really helpful to see how these physical problems can affect you emotionally and psychologically.

In Chinese medicine, the liver is sometimes described as something like a military commander in the body. It formulates tactics and strategies, moving blood and energy (qi) throughout the body.

As we have learned, the thyroid is part of the endocrine system which is viewed as qi and is derived from the yang energy of the kidneys.

So the ancient Chinese recognized this relationship and how important one is for the other.

The liver needs that qi to have the energy to do its job, and if it is clogged or blocked it can't facilitate the movement of that energy throughout the body. When the liver gets stuck or clogged, the most common emotion that people experience is anger.

This can be directed outwardly at people you know (usually people closest to you: family, co-workers, or friends) or this anger can be directed inwardly and result in depression and feeling of self-hatred and low self-worth.

Or sometimes you have a combination of these two.

In fact, depression is one of the most common symptoms associated with Hashimoto's and anti-depressants are some of the most commonly prescribed drugs for people with hypothyroid issues.

The Gall Bladder

The Gall Bladder, the yang organ of the wood element, stores and secretes bile, this stimulates flow through the stomach and intestines and is very important in helping us to absorb and eliminate different foods as well as different ideas and concepts.

So proper bile flow and production also help us with proper judgment, clear thinking and decision making.

If there are Liver/Gall Bladder issues we can end up taking actions without thinking them through, or making decisions and not following through on them or simply getting stuck, unable to decide what to do.

According to Deke Kendall, in his book the Dao of Chinese Medicine, the endocrine gland associated with the wood element is the pineal gland.

He makes the connection via the spirit of the liver which is called the hun, in Chinese.

Functional activities in the liver, like the breakdown of carbs, fats and protein are influenced by natural cycles in the body.

Many metabolic activities in the liver are inhibited at night and then reactivated the next morning by daylight.

These events are now known to be controlled by melatonin, the hormone produced by the pineal gland that is made from central serotonin.

Central serotonin levels have a direct influences on our moods. If you have too much melatonin or a diet low in trytophan which is a precursor to serotonin, you may develop symptoms like depression, an inability to concentrate, mental fatigue, PMS, carb cravings, obesity, reduced libido, and chronic pain.

Many of these disorders mentioned above are worse for people who live in higher northern or southern latitudes where there is less sunlight.

The pineal gland sets the body's internal clock based on light. The liver's sense organ is the eyes, perhaps that is the connection.

Clinical pearl: It's also interesting to note that melatonin rhythm has its own internal clock that has monthly or lunar cycle and it may influence hormones released by the hypothalamus.

Taking melatonin as a supplement can disrupt natural cortisol rhythms and can actually disrupt sleep patterns.

Another interesting thing to note about melatonin is that it is a TH1 stimulant and some people with TH1 dominance can have flare ups of their symptoms at night, especially during the hours of 1:00 AM and 5:00 AM when melatonin peaks.

The Liver's Impact on the Body's Internal Environment

The environmental condition associated with the wood element is wind. In nature wind moves in an unpredictable fashion.

When external events are rapidly changing, the facility of the liver and gall bladder are to make decisions and implement plans so that we can adapt to our circumstances.

If the wood element is out of balance, and we habitually react in anger, then we might develop internal wind.

Symptoms of internal wind are usually neurological, like convulsions, muscle twitches and spasms, headaches, or pains that change location rapidly.

Emotionally, wind can become anger that blows up like a storm whenever we are faced with a surprise change or unexpected circumstance.

This can result in indecisiveness and poor planning that make it difficult for us to put together a coherent plan of action.

So anger, like wind can confuse your vision and make it difficult to overcome life's challenges.

On the other hand, if you suppress your anger this may cause stagnation as resentment builds up inside of you.

Kindness Is Key to Healing the Wood Element

One of my favorite expressions about resentment is that it is like taking poison and waiting for the other person (the person you resent) to die.

What this ultimately does, is stop you from growing. Because everything that is an obstacle or that is unexpected makes you angry and this distracts you from adapting and moving forward.

In some ways, the opposite of that anger is benevolence and kindness. When we can see events from that point of view, we are able to see the big picture of how external circumstances complement our own internal plans.

The sage is the enlightened being, he or she moves through life in a calm unattached manner, not controlled by their emotions.

This detachment allows us to not blame ourselves or anyone else. This is when life starts to fire on all cylinders. Now the gall bladder can manifest the inner plan and read external events appropriately so that everything lines up.

It's a beautiful thing.

The Life of A Sage: They Forget the Liver

There was a famous sage named Chuan Tzu and here's how he describes the life of the sage…

"They forget the liver and gall, cast aside eyes and ears, turning and revolving, ending and beginning again, unaware of where they start or finish.

Idly, they roam beyond dust and dirt; they wander free and easy in the service of inaction..."

There is a concept in Taoism called wu wei (pronounced wu way), which can be translated to "doing without doing". It all becomes that effortless.

311

Man, that's what I want!

Wu wei for days!

So, to summarize: it really comes down to this. Do you want to be right or do you want to be happy?

The habitual reaction of anger drives the liver and gall bladder to either under or overuse their natural creativity in directing the process of growth. You never feel fulfilled because everything becomes an obstacle that just feeds your anger.

Or you feel so defeated by every challenge that you just give up and don't make any progress.

Only when you can feel love and kindness for yourself and others can that natural wood energy flow.

Wu wei, all the way!

Let it go. Love yourself then you can love others, and then it just flows.

That takes practice. It really does.

And that's where we're going to leave it. Just wu wei.

Effortless doing without doing.

Try to imagine living your life like that.

Or better yet, start living your life like that and see what happens.

Chapter Twenty-Four

Using the A.P.A.R.T. System to Heal the Wood Element

The A.P.A.R.T. System

1. A = Ask and Asses

Your journal should be filling up by now. This time, look for symptoms of problems with the Wood Eement. Note what they are, then create a plan for addressing them. After that, you must act on your plan. Follow through and do what you have planned.

After that take inventory of what you did. Look at what worked and what didn't. Both will provide valuable information.

Double down on what worked, change what didn't. Once a year, during the spring, revisit healing the Wood Element.

Gallbladder and Liver -Wood Symptoms

Gall Bladder:

Greasy or high-fat foods cause distress
Lower bowel gas and/or bloating several hours after eating
Bitter metallic taste in mouth, especially in the morning
Unexplained itchy skin
Yellowish cast to eyes
Stool color alternates from clay colored to normal brown
Reddened skin, especially palms
Dry or flaky skin and/or hair
History of gallbladder attacks or stones
Have you had your gallbladder removed?

Liver Detoxification:

Acne and unhealthy skin
Excessive hair loss
Overall sense of bloating
Bodily swelling for no reason
Hormone imbalances
Weight gain
Poor bowel function
Excessively foul-smelling sweat

Symptoms of Liver Imbalance in Chinese Medicine

Emotions of the Wood Element: One of the most common signs of disharmony of the liver is symptoms related to anger. Rage, being short tempered, mean, cruel, sadistic, easily frustrated, rude, impatient, arrogant or flying off the handle at the slightest provocation can all be examples of a dysfunctional liver.

It's no accident that drinking alcohol can often accompany these emotions because alcohol is toxic to the liver and must be metabolized and detoxified. Often times this kind of behavior is followed by guilt, self loathing, depression and excessive self criticism, as well. And this is another manifestation of this energy turned inward.

Common Syndromes of the Liver

Liver Stagnation: Excesses of one kind or another are a common with the liver. Too much eating, especially greasy fried foods, too much alcohol, and too much sugar can all clog the liver and cause significant health problems.

Since the liver is the conductor of blood and energy flow in the body, one of the consequences of these excesses can be cysts and lumps throughout the body. These can found anywhere, but are sometimes found in the thyroid.

We've seen the important connections between the liver and the thyroid.
When the liver is stagnant, a lump may be felt in the throat, even though one cannot physically be found; when a goiter exists (an enlarged thyroid, visible as a swelling at the front in the neck), this may also a sign of a congested liver.

The chest or abdomen may also become distended, or breasts enlarged. Swelling or lumps can occur in the neck, groin, sides of the body, and the lateral portion of the thighs.

The Liver Also Rules the Tendons and Eyes

When there is too little energy and blood flow in the body , then the tendons are not nourished and can easily become compromised. In fact, many tendon issues are not caused by swelling, but rather tears and fraying of the tendons. This is often the cause of tendon pain in conditions like Carpal Tunnel Syndrome or Lateral Epicondylitis (Tennis elbow).

In fact, it's really interesting to note that a recent review in the Muscles, Ligaments and Tendons Journal found that there are thyroid receptors in tendons and that thyroid hormone plays an important role in keeping tendons healthy and strong.

This is yet another interesting connection related to Hashimoto's, Carpal tunnel syndrome and other tendon related issues are very common.

It is not clear why this is true. One theory is that myxedema could impact the median nerve sheath and lead to compression and impairment of the nerve. Hypothyroidism, because of its impact on peripheral vascular flow can lead to poor nourishment of tendons and may also cause just this type of problem.

In fact, in my opinion, every patient who is diagnosed with carpal tunnel should have a thyroid work up to rule out thyroid disease.

Another common issue that is related to the liver are eye conditions. The eyes become inflamed, swollen, or pulled out of focus by the muscles that control them.

Much like the tendons, the eyes rely on small capillaries and blood flow for their health and nourishment.

Thyroid eye disease is also very common and while Graves is more often associated with eye issues, Hashimoto's patients also often suffer from serious eye problems. It was my own eye issues that lead to my initial diagnosis.

Many eye conditions such as glaucoma, macular degeneration, cataracts, red, dry eyes, near and far sightedness are thought to be related to the condition of the liver.

Corneal disease has been found in Wilson's disease, in cirrhosis, hepatitis and more. Glaucoma has been identified in liver diseases such as Maroteaux Lamy and Scheie's syndrome. Vitamin A deficiency and problems with the rods of the retina have been noted in billiary cirrhosis. Other issues involving the optic and cranial nerves have also been linked to liver diseases.

One treatment strategy for eye issues is to heal and detoxify the liver. In fact, many writers and therapists who teach vision correction suggest a dietary method that uses this approach.

This strategy includes a vegetarian diet, with an emphasis on fresh raw vegetables and sprouts. Meals are small and eating the last meal in the evening is recommended.

Eating moderate amounts of food and avoiding late meals can allow the liver and gallbladder time to prepare for regeneration during the time that the energy of the body circulates through them. According to Chinese Medicine this is from11:00 pm to 3:00 am.

In addition, the B vitamin known as folic acid is considered an important nutrient in the treatment and correction of mypoia. Folic acid is found in green leafy vegetables and sprouts.

Liver Blood Issues

As we saw the liver is an important filter in the body. In Chinese medicine the liver is also thought to store and purify the blood. When the liver is clogged and full of fatty tissue (as it is in metabolic syndrome which is caused by eating too much sugar) then toxins can build up.

This build up of toxins in the blood is thought to cause of acne, eczema, carbuncles, boil, and even some allergies. And, as we saw when looked at detoxification in the liver, problems with phase II can lead to the build up of highly toxic substances in the body. And these can contribute to degenerative disease and disease of inflammation like autoimmune disease and cancer.

This is precisely why healthy phase I and phase II detoxification is so important for many of the body's other systems.

Testing: Cholesterol, LDL, triglycerides can be important indicators of both sugar metabolism and hypothyroidism. If these are high, your HDL is low and you're eating a "perfect diet" it could be it's not so perfect when it comes to sugar or it could be hypothyroidism. Or, of course, it could be both.

Liver Enzymes: AST, ALT, GGT

High or low liver enzymes can both be problems. Elevations mean inflammation of the liver, low enzymes may mean deficiencies in important vitamins such as vitamin B6.

2. P = Prioritize and Plan

Not everything has the same level importance. This is what 80/20 teaches us. Some things are having more of an impact than others. Figure out which they are (the positive feedback loops) and then make a plan to fix them.

The liver's importance in many metabolic functions and in the conversion of thyroid hormone makes it a priority in virtually everyone. There really is no downside in improving liver health and function.

3. A = Act and Adapt

Act and put your plan into motion. Then observe what the results are. Double down on what works and change what doesn't. And results should be apparent relatively quickly. If they aren't you need to make changes.

An excellent time to work on detoxifying the liver is during the elimination phase of the Autoimmune Paleo diet. This provides the perfect opportunity to give your liver a break from sugar, processed foods and other toxins that enter the diet via our food supply.

Foods:

Foods which stimulate the liver and relieve stagnation -watercress, all members of the onion family, mustard greens, turmeric, basil, bay leaf, cardamom, marjoram, cumin, fennel, dill, ginger, black pepper, horseradish, rosemary, various mints, beets, taro root, sweet rice, amasake, strawberry, peach ,cherry, chestnut, pine nut, cabbage, turnip root, kohlrabi, cauliflower, broccoli, and brussels sprouts

-**Raw foods**- sprouted grains, beans, and seeds, fresh vegetables and fruits

-**Foods which harmonize the liver**- Honey, Honey mixed with apple cider, and licorice root. (We've discussed the many problems that sugar can cause, so be cautious with sugar of any kind)

-**Bitter and sour foods reduce excesses of the liver**- Vinegar- apple cider, brown rice, rice wine, lemon, lime or grapefruit, rye, romaine lettuce, asparagus, amaranth, quinoa, alfalfa, radish leaves, and citrus peel

-**Foods for detoxifying and cooling the liver**- Mung beans and their sprouts, celery, seaweed, lettuce, cucumber, watercress, tofu, millet, plum, chlorophyll rich foods

-**Reducing toxicity resulting from overconsumption of meat**- Mushrooms, rhubarb root or stem, radish, and daikon radish

-**Deficient liver blood**- Spirulina, chlorophyll rich foods, dark grape, blackberries, huckleberries, raspberries, black strap molasses

-**Foods which accelerate liver rejuvenation**- spirulina, wild blue green, chlorella, parsley, kale, watercress, alfalfa, collard greens

-**Gallbladder cleanse**- parsnips, seaweeds, lemons, lines, turmeric, radish(removes deposits and stones from the gallbladder), lemon juice, olive oil

Common Liver/Gall Bladder Issues

PMS (Premenstrual Syndrome): In Chinese medicine this is seen as a disorder of the blood. Either stagnant blood, too little blood (anemia), heat in the blood and stagnation of liver energy.

Foods for PMS: At least one week prior to onset of symptoms eat ginger, green onions, fennel, orange peel, spinach, walnuts, hawthorn berries, cinnamon, back pepper, Chinese dates, Dang gui

Gallstones: Cornsilk, water chestnuts, seaweed, beet tops, watermelon, celery, watercress, winter melon, watermelon rind, winter melon rind, green tea powder, distilled water – also one of the most important things to do to prevent gall stones is to ensure that you have proper stomach acid levels.

Herbs for Liver/Gall Bladder

-**Stimulate liver out of stagnancy:** lemon balm, angelica root, prickly ash bark,

-**Bitter herbs-** dandelion root, bupleurum, milk thistle seeds, Oregon grape fruit, chamomile flowers

-**Herbs for building yin in blood-** flax oil, extracted oils of borage, evening primrose, black current seeds, aloe vera gel

-**Herbs for deficient liver blood-** Dang gui root, prepared rehmannia root, peony root, yellow dock root

-**Gallbladder cleanse-** Cleavers, chamomile tea

Other herbs that are helpful for the liver:

Ginger: this common food contains chemicals that have been shown to increase bile secretion and to reduce cholesterol levels by up regulating an enzyme responsible for bile acid production (cholesterol-7-alpha-hydorxylase).

Dandelion: The root of this common weed promotes the production of bile and its delivery to the gall bladder. It causes the gall bladder to contract and release bile.

Milk Thistle: This herb increases the solubility of bile and has been shown to significantly lower cholesterol concentrations in the gall bladder. It has potent anti-oxidant activity which supports detoxification and it prevents depletion of glutathione in the liver, which is often depleted in people with Hashimoto's. It also has anti-inflammatory properties and it promotes protein synthesis to replace damaged liver cells.

Panax ginseng: This herb has been shown in several studies to have numerous positive impacts on liver function. It has been shown to reverse fatty liver in animals and can be really helpful in cleaning toxins out of the liver. It also has really important benefits for the immune system like promoting Kupffer cells (specialized immune cells located in the liver) and can be beneficial in balancing the immune system by increasing key proteins like IL-8.

Herba sargassi, Laminaria Kun Bu: These seaweeds have important detoxification properties and can be used to treat metabolic toxicosis with arthritis, rheumatism, dermatitis and psoriasis. They are quite mild and have very few if any side effects. In addition, they are rich in trace minerals and are helpful in reducing swelling, particularly in the lymphatic glands.

A word of caution with seaweeds: They contain iodine which can be problematic with some people with Hashimoto's.

Fructus Gardeniae: This herb is the seed pod of the gardenia plant. It has potent anti-bacterial and anti-viral properties and can be used to reduce liver and gallblader congestion and infections.

Caution: Liver infections can be quite serious, consult a trained physician if you suspect that you have any form of hepatitis or liver disease.

Rhubarb Root: This herb is a potent laxative that can be used to treat acute gall bladder and pancreatic infections. It has potent anti-bacterial, anti-fungal and anti-viral properties.

Dosage is critical with this herb and too much can cause gastric pain and diarrhea. Never use during pregnancy or lactation or with gout, hemorrhoids or oxalic acid stones. Consult a trained professional before using this herb.

Qi Gong for the Wood Element
Twist and Release

Twist and release

This exercise is benefical for the whole body. It's effective in relieving tension and lowering blood pressure. In traditional Chinese medicine, twisting the waist helps balance the yin and yang energies in the body, it's soothing to the heart and it increasing breathing capacity.

Because this is focused on the Wood Element, it can also be effective in releasing pent up anger and aggression.

Begin by standing in the natural standing form, feet shoulder width apart, weight evenly distributed and knees slightly bent. To make the exercise more of a challenge bend the knees more deeply and widen the stance slightly. It's more important that you can relax in the posture, so only goes as far as you can and stay relaxed.

Place your hands over your thighs with your fingers pointing inward and your thumbs grasping the outside of the leg.

Put the focus of your mind down to the bottom of your feet. Relax your hips and wrists.

Next, inhale, rotate your torso to the left, leading with the left shoulder. Then look back to the right and over the right shoulder to the ground looking down towards the right foot. If you need to, you can lower the right shoulder a bit, but try not to hunch forward or pull backwards.

As you shift your focus to the right and back, imagine a string pulling your head up and slightly back.

Arch your upper back to get an additional stretch. It is ok to lift the heel of your right foot off the ground but remember to keep both knees bent the whole time. And keep your hands on your thighs the whole time.

At the end of the movement hold the pose for a second or two.

At first, this movement may seem a bit awkward, but try to keep the movements smooth and do it in one flowing sequence. Stay relaxed and flexible, avoid tightening the hips and waist. As you exhale, bend the right knee and turn back to the starting position.

repeat the whole movement on the opposite side.
*Repeat 3 times on each side, 1 or 2 times per day.

Want to see a video demonstration of this qi gong exercise? Visit the supplemental page on our website:
https://hashimotos-diet.com/roadmap-to-remission-supplemental/

4. R= Reassess and Readjust

Retest, Reassess and ask all over again. Figure out what worked and what didn't. Double down on what worked and either eliminate or recreate a plan for what didn't.

The liver and wood element is constantly under assault in today's world. Revisiting the liver and periodically supporting and cleansing it is an excellent general principle.

Springtime is the best time to do this. Doing a gentle liver cleanse each spring is a great way to "clean house" in your body regularly.

5. T = Try and Try Again

Keep doing it, keep refining, keep building on the positive results and keep looking for the remaining positive feedback loops that are causing vicious cycles.
Remember that the positive attributes of the Wood Element are kindness and compassion. As you travel on this journey of healing always remember to be kind and have compassion for everyone, including yourself.

Chapter Twenty-Five

The Fire Element

This is a really interesting pairing in Chinese medicine. We saw with the metal element that 2 apparently unrelated systems actually had a lot of connections (in that case via the lymphatic system).

Well, with the heart and small intestine the connection is clearly via the cardiovascular system.

Look at the anatomical drawing that we've used for this chapter. See at all the vascular activity? The greatest number of arterial vessels supplies the small intestines. Why is there so much?

Well, as every grade school child knows: the heart's job is to pump blood to all of the organs, tissues, and cells in your body through blood vessels (arteries and veins). This is really important because blood delivers the oxygen and nutrients that every cell needs and removes dangerous wastes.

Well, where do those nutrients come from? Most of them come from the small intestines.

The small intestine is the part of the intestines where 90% of the digestion and absorption of food occurs, the other 10% taking place in the stomach and large intestine. The main function of the small intestine is absorption of nutrients and minerals from food.

The Heart

The heart circulates those nutrients by pumping blood throughout the body. When blood is pumped through your body, it puts pressure against the walls of your blood vessels.

Right? This is your blood pressure.

When doctors describe blood pressure, they use two numbers like "120 over 70". These numbers describe the pressure when your heart pumps blood into your blood vessels (the high number) and the pressure when your heart relaxes (the low number).

Imagine squeezing a ketchup bottle. When you squeeze it to 'pump' ketchup onto your plate, the pressure is high. When you stop squeezing, the pressure is low.

Blood pressure can change a lot during the day. It is usually lower while you are relaxing and higher when you are active. Other things like pregnancy, smoking, medication, being stressed and thyroid hormone levels can change your blood pressure.

Hypothyroid, But High Blood Pressure?

Usually, with hypothyroid conditions, you're blood pressure is low and with hyperthyroid conditions it tends to be high. But there are many reasons why this is not always the case, in fact, many Hashimoto's people actually have high blood pressure.

This is because even though many thyroid patients, or those being treated with T4 meds like Synthroid, can start out with low blood pressure, factors related to having functional hypothyroidism can actually create hypertension and high blood pressure over time.

For example, as we saw when we looked at the Water Element hypothyroidism leads to a host of problems physiologically that cause kidney and cardiovascular problems.

For example, there's less blood flow to the kidneys, this causes the kidneys to not filter waste products like creatinine from your body properly.

In addition, when your blood pressure is low, and "angiotensin" is produced, this raises your blood pressure.

Also when you are hypothyroid, blood is taken from the extremities into the body, which tends to raise pressure by forcing the same volume of blood into a smaller network of vessels.

This process is brought about by a constriction of peripheral vessels. Hypothyroid patients produce an excess of noradrenalin from the adrenal gland, which constricts blood vessels all over the body, another effort of the body to deal with the low blood pressure.

This in turn is partly related to the effort by the body to raise blood sugar levels when low. We've already discussed this, as well.

These problems may or may not be caused by being overmedicated. Anxiety, tachycardia (fast heart rate), and high blood pressure that people with Hashimoto's experience is not always from being hyperthyroid or overmedicated, it may also be from noradrenaline that the body is secreting for energy to compensate for the lack of thyroid hormone.

Unfortunately, what often happens is that they're prescribed blood pressure medications (such as beta blockers) and/or anti-anxiety medications (such as benzodiazepines).

Neither of these drugs corrects the underlying functional hypothyroidism (low thyroid condition) that caused the symptoms in the first place, and both have side effects. In one study, noradrenaline was three times higher in hypothyroid subjects than normal controls when lying down.

So what was once low blood pressure, now takes a nasty turn towards hypertension, or high blood pressure.

Another....you guessed it, **vicious cycle**.

Obviously, too high blood pressure can be dangerous. It means that there is too much stress on your blood vessels. This makes the vessels weak and can damage them. Imagine squeezing a ketchup bottle really hard and fast until it breaks. High blood pressure is a major cause of heart disease.

How the Thyroid Impacts Cardiovascular Function

Ok, so let's take a look at how else the thyroid impacts cardiovascular function. Firstly, thyroid hormone has a direct impact on cholesterol; with hypothyroidism serum cholesterol increases.

Thyroid hormone stimulates an enzyme called HMG-CoA reductase, the same enzyme that statin drugs inhibit. This speeds up the synthesis and utilization of cholesterol by the body.

Thyroid hormone stimulates the removal of cholesterol by the liver using LDL receptors. In a hypothyroid state, this whole process is slowed and the result is that cholesterol builds up and isn't cleared as quickly.

Hypothryoidism can also cause homocysteine levels to rise. High homocysteine can lead to inflammation of the arteries and can make you more prone to blood clots, heart attacks and strokes.

We talked about that in the last chapter too, because nourishing certain pathways in the liver can really help bring down high homocysteine.

CRP another risk factor and inflammatory marker for inflammation in the arteries is also often high with hypothyroidism.

Another odd thing that too little thyroid hormone can cause is lower plasma volume. This is caused by capillaries becoming more permeable and when this happens albumin and water leak into the interstitial spaces.

Albumin and water leaking into these spaces causes swelling from edema and water retention, often in your ankles or lower legs.

So here again, we have the makings of a particular dangerous vicious cycle. In the chapter on the Earth Element, we spoke about how blood sugar problems like metabolic syndrome can create a lot of conditions that make you more likely to develop heart disease.

Well, when you combine that with hypothyroidism, you have a very potent combination that can put you at risk for heart attack and stroke.

Thyroid Hormone and The Heart

Another area that does not get the attention it deserves is the impact of thyroid hormone on the heart and cardiac tissue. One of the things that research is starting to reveal is that thyroid hormone is absorbed differently by different tissues of the body.

In other words not every part of you body is affected the same way by T4 and T3. For example, the pituitary is different than every cell in the body with different deiodinase enzymes and it has more sensitive to thyroid hormone receptors.

Many physicans assume, incorrectly, that thyroid hormone is simply absorbed via diffusion (which is basically like the cell sucking hormone in through a biochemical straw). However the reality is that the process is energy dependent and called active transport which means it requires the body to use energy to push it into the cells.

In addition, different parts of the body respond differently to T3 and T4. 90% of T3 is absorbed by the stomach while T4 is much less efficient (50-90%) and T4 requires much more energy to get absorbed.

T3 affects cardiac muscle cell (myocytes), contraction of the heart, it also impacts the performance of sodium, potassium, and calcium channels in the heart. What this means is that just throwing more thyroid hormone at the problem may not be the answer and can have unintended consequences.

Something else the research has identified is that thyroid autoimmunity can affect the valves of the heart. So, if you have Hashimoto's and have been diagnosed with heart murmur, an echocardiogram might be a really good idea.

Again, showing…Jeez…I feel like a broken record sometimes, but I have to say it… how important it is to deal with this problem from multiple directions. We must treat all these different systems.

CASE STUDY: HEALING THE HEART

Here's a perfect example of a case that represents the healing the Fire Element quite well. (Used with permission)

Patient is a 75 year old female with Hashimoto's who presented with many cardiovascular symptoms including palpitations in the morning, an irregular heartbeat, constipation, sensitivity on her scalp and back of head, and red itchy eyes in the morning.

Laboratory testing revealed an elevated TSH, low T4, low T3 and free T3, high cholesterol, high homocysteine, and hypertension. Her cardiologist also had done a workup and it revealed Atrial fibrillation.

She had recently undergone chelation therapy due to her practitioner finding high levels of lead and pesticides in her body.

We worked to heal her gut and support her liver detoxification pathways. Gave her plenty of anti-inflammatories and glutathione. Got her on a strict Autoimmune Paleo diet.

In addition, we worked to improve thyroid hormone conversion and absorption and to get her TSH into normal range. We also supplemented with B vitamins to bring down the homocysteine levels.

Here is a real email she sent us 6 months later:

"I just came home from the cardiologist, got tested and received a clean bill of health. Yep, he said that everything with my heart is normal and I don't need to come back! This, after continual Afibbs and suggestion of beta blockers, blood thinners and possible ablation (going into my heart to desensitize trigger tissue).

Marc, your course influenced me and gave me courage to walk your talk. I can't thank you enough for your help in turning my life around."

PS: I found a new friend (I'm not kidding). The name is Hashimoto's. It knows my body better than anything else. It guides to healthy eating and healthy living. It is always beside me, watching over me. And when I stray, it gently pushes me onto the right path. But if I don't listen - it has a strong voice - for my own good. What a pal. I'm blessed."
Edith S., Maine

Again, we can't promise these results to everyone, but Edith deserves the credit for following our plan, really following through and making the changes she needed to make.

She also was able to change her thinking about this disease and was actually able to see some blessing in it. That's truly inspirational to me to see that someone at that age could be open to growing and changing.

Here is some additional commentary she added:

"So this is what I did:

Foremost I kept in mind the most important thing (in my opinion) something you said in your webinar, don't listen to test numbers, but listen to how you FEEL. Wow, to me that was big!

I felt that I did not want a disease label slapped on me! And for life?! No way! I'm going to get BALANCED! One organ at a time. My heart to me was most crucial. So I went to town. Yeah, I tried everything. If it didn't work, I dismissed it.

All summer I worked on the Paleo diet. Triggers were eliminated. My brain cleared up, perhaps since I'm mashing in Rosemary into my sweet potatoes, as well as Tumeric every day.

My sore scalp disappeared when by accident I forgot all my vitamins. I had an overload of vitamins because I was getting them from the healthy (everything organic and colorful variety) foods.

I truly had to adjust my years of conditioning to think a certain way. My body was craving food every two hours. So I said, your desire is my command. I fed it (only healthy, organic) on demand, no questions asked or contemplated . After a while it told me, enough already! And now I'm eating normal because I respect my body when it gives me a signal.

Seems like it enjoys ginger (freshly grated) tea about half an hour after I eat. So I keep a batch at hand (no plastic jars, only glass). I don't take fish oil in capsules, felt an overload of swallowing the outer capsule. Take cod liver oil instead (with lemon flavor). Not bad. Also take a condensed berry extract (anthocyanin) and lecithin."

Wow! Notice how she really learned to listen to her body and trust what she heard (all at age 75). Totally awesome!

Anemia, No Bueno

Another area that is of concern with Hashimoto's is anemia. There are a number of theories about why this is.

> **One thing that research has revealed is that T4 concentrations are connected to hemoglobin levels.**

So with less T4, there is less oxygen being carried to the peripheral tissues. We also know that the anemia of hypothyroidism is caused by a decrease in erythropoiesis or the creating of red blood cells in the marrow.

Other anemias include iron deficiency anemia. This may be caused by blood loss (during the cycle) or more often by what we discussed in the Chapters on the Earth Element, low stomach acid levels - caused by hypothyroidism.

B12 and folate deficiency are also possible, with absorption being reduced by the same cause . Both T4 and B12 therapy may be helpful.

Another fact, which I mentioned in the Chapters on the Metal Element, is that once you have one autoimmune disease, it's not that hard to develop others and about 10 to 12% of Hashimoto's patients also have pernicious anemia.

This is an autoimmune disease that causes low B12 levels usually caused by the destruction of gastric parietal cells (and autoantibody inactivation of intrinsic factor) which is required for B12 absorption.

Thyroid hormone and B12 supplementation are both important here as well.

Bleeding problems can also occur with hypothyroidism. This can lead to bruising easily, prolonged bleeding when injured, or heavy bleeding during the cycle.

Clinical pearl: Hypothryoidism can also make bleeding after taking aspirin or other NSAIDS (Non Steroidal Anti-Inflammatory Drugs like ibuprophen, acetaminophen, aspirin and Naproxen, etc.) more intense, another reason to be very careful about NSAID use when you have Hashimoto's.

This is something that it is recommended to avoid when doing the elimination diet. These drugs are not that safe to begin with, but when combined with a hypothyroid state, you can have real serious problems.

OK, that's a lot of heart and blood related stuff that we just covered.

Recap

1. Hypothyroidism can cause high blood pressure. This can be caused by the kidneys and the adrenals. Both of which we looked at in the Water Element.

2. Hypothyroidism can impact cholesterol break down and utilization and can cause high cholesterol.

3. It can also cause high homocysteine, and high CRP (C reactive protein). The combined effect of high blood pressure, high cholesterol and high homocysteine and high CRP means that you may be at a major risk for a heart attack or a stroke. Not good.

4. Hashimoto's can also lead to various anemias: iron deficiency, B12 deficiency, pernicious anemia (another autoimmune disease) and excessive bleeding.

Holy smokes, do you see how this is so much more than a thyroid disorder? And do you see why I wanted to write this book?

I hope so. And I hope you are working with someone and following a similar plan to what we are advocating because everything we have looked at and the treatment approach we have shared is one that addresses all these different areas of the body.

For example, as you have seen, we recommend limiting the additional causes of high cholesterol by dealing with blood sugar imbalances, reducing inflammation wherever possible, reducing stress and it's corrosive effects.

Here's a little secret. The goal of this book and the process we are describing is not just to get your Hashimoto's into remission.

Our goal is to help you keep it there and to provide you with a blueprint for happiness and longevity, so that you can enjoy life again and be there for your friends and family.

I wish that for you.

Chapter Twenty-Six

The Small Intestines:
Ground Zero

Ok, so now, let's look a little more closely at the small intestine.

Digestion involves two distinct parts. The first is mechanical digestion by chewing, grinding, churning and mixing that takes place in the mouth and the stomach. We looked at that in the Earth Element and saw how important stomach acid was for this.

The second part of digestion is the chemical digestion that uses enzymes, bile acids etc. in order to break down food material into a form that can then be absorbed, then assimilated into the tissues of the body. Chemical digestion occurs mostly in the small intestine.

Enzymes such as trypsin and chymotrypsin, secreted by the pancreas, act upon proteins, peptides and amino acids. This breaks them down to smaller peptides. Chemical breakdown begins in the stomach and continues until the large intestine.

Enzymes, like lipases also secreted from the pancreas, act on fats and lipids in diet. This breaks the triglycerides into free fatty acids and monoglycerides.

It is helped by bile salts secreted by the liver and the gall bladder. The lipase is soluble in water but the fatty triglycerides are not.

The bile salts hold the triglycerides in the watery environment until the lipase can break them into the smaller parts that can enter the intestinal lining (villi) for absorption.

Carbohydrates are broken down to simple sugars and monosaccharides like glucose. Pancreatic amylase breaks down some carbohydrates to oligosaccharides as well.

(Some carbohydrates and fibers pass undigested to the large intestine where they may, depending on their type, be broken-down by intestinal bacteria. This is where FODMAP comes into play. Remember we covered that earlier in the Chapter on the Earth Element)

Once broken down the nutrients are absorbed by the inner walls of the small intestine into the blood stream. The nutrients are rendered small enough so that they may pass, or "be transported", across the epithelial cells of the gastrointestinal tract into the blood.

The small intestine is good for absorption since it has a large inner surface area. This is done by the villi and microvilli. **These are what is damaged with leaky gut.**

Small Intestines Are Important for Absorbing Everything

Approximately 80% of water is absorbed by the small intestine, 10% by the large intestine and the remaining 10% excreted in the feces.

All of the important electrolytes are absorbed in the small intestine: chloride, iodine, calcium (these are absorbed with the help of vitamin D), iron, magnesium and potassium.

Vitamins including fat soluble ones (Vitamins A, D, E and K) are absorbed together with dietary fats.

Water soluble vitamins like vitamins B and C are absorbed by diffusion. Vitamin B12 combined with intrinsic factor (from the stomach) is absorbed by active transport.

Of these iron is absorbed in the duodenum, most are absorbed in the jejunum and Vitamin B12 and bile salts are absorbed in the later part of the ileum.

Ok, so how does this relate to Hashimoto's?

Well, if you remember back in the Chapters on the Metal Element, a lot of the lymphatic system is located in and around the small intestines, just as a lot of the arterial blood supply is there.

So, when we have leaky gut, a lot of foreign matter can end up in your blood stream that shouldn't be there. This causes a massive immune response.

The Small Intestine is Ground Zero for Autoimmunity

Dr. Alessio Fasano, MD, an expert on the origins of autoimmunity has found the cause of this disease in the intestines. In a paper published in the Clinical Review of Allergy Immunology February 2012 , he noted that,

"Together with the gut-associated lymphoid tissue and the neuroendocrine network, the intestinal epithelial barrier, with its intercellular tight junctions, controls the equilibrium between tolerance and immunity to non-self antigens. Zonulin is the only physiologic modulator of intercellular tight junctions described so far that is involved in trafficking of macromolecules and, therefore, in tolerance/immune response balance. When the zonulin pathway is deregulated in genetically susceptible individuals, autoimmune disorders can occur."

What that means in plain English is that the breakdown of the barrier of the intestines is the pathway to autoimmune disease.

We've already looked at the Metal and Earth Elements and we discussed how both are involved in autoimmunity. And we also discovered zonulin, "the zipper" of the intestinal walls.

A leaky gut or damaged intestine has been found in every autoimmune disease that has been tested including rheumatoid arthritis, ankylosing spondylitis, inflammatory bowel disease (Crohn's disease and ulcerative colitis), celiac disease, multiple sclerosis, type I diabetes and, yes, Hashimoto's.

In the small intestine this damage leads to immune system stimulation, the wrong types of things in the blood stream and, ultimately, a systemic problem that results in the loss of self-tolerance.

This means that the immune system gets so overwhelmed it can't tell what our tissue is and what a foreign invader is.

SIBO: Small Intestine Bacterial Overgrowth

Another serious issue that we touched on earlier in the book was SIBO.

Unlike FODMAP, which sounds like a bad corporation, this one sounds like a good charity, doesn't it?

"Please give to SIBO. We understand the plight of the small intestine, we care. Give generously today and save the ecosystem that gives you life."

You may recall that SIBO stands for Small Intestine Bacterial Overgrowth.

This can be making your Hashimoto's worse because bacterial gut infections constantly activate the immune system, which can make it difficult to manage the autoimmune part of this party.

Which Came First Leaky Gut or SIBO?

There are many causes of the breakdown of the intestines.

These include NSAID use, alcohol, gluten and other dietary proteins, bacterial overgrowth, environmental toxins and more.

And once this breaks down it alters the whole ecosystem of the gut.
It's hard to know which came first.

And at the end of the day, it doesn't really matter.

What matters is what causes it and what we can do to heal it.

Symptoms of SIBO

SIBO has a number of possible symptoms, but mostly these involve bloating, gas, diarrhea and/or constipation.

The hallmark symptom is bloating and discomfort after eating certain foods.

Basically here's what happens: The wrong type of bacteria end up getting into the small intestine. They migrate from the large intestine and take over.

They feed on certain types of foods like sugars, galactans, fructans and starch.

In reality, SIBO should be considered with abdominal discomfort after eating any of the following things:

– Starches
– Sugars/fructose
– Fructans
– Prebiotics
– Probiotics
– Fiber supplements
– Rice or pea powder from metabolic powders
– Galactans

You may notice that many of the foods listed here can also aggravate candida. And sometimes candida is blamed for what is actually SIBO.

5 Main Causes of SIBO

The causes of SIBO matter because when we understand the causes, we can figure out how to fix them.

These include:

1. Too little stomach acid.

Hashimoto's and hypothyroidism leads to lower production of gastrin and stomach acid. This is super common. We learned about this in the section on the Earth Element.

Unfortunately, many people develop GERD or acid reflux and are prescribed proton pump inhibitors and antacids that just make everything worse.

2. An immune suppressed gut.

Many factors can lead to immune suppression in the gut. 2 important ones are long term corticosteroid treatment and chronic stress.

In either case, a lot of cortisol or corticosteroids cause the immune system to shut down and can contribute to leaky gut. This results in poor defenses and systemic immune activation.

With Hashimoto's the body is under a great deal of physiological stress, all the time. Therefore, extra emotional stress and abnormally stressful events often result in people getting a lot sicker.

This is one of the reasons why.

3. Injury to the gut nervous system (known as the ENS or enteric nervous system)

The gut has been called the body's "second brain" because it has its own nervous system and produces many of the neurotransmitters that are also produced in the brain.

Well, just like our other brain this can degenerate and break down with age and with diseases like chronic celiac disease, sceleroderma and IBS.

And just like neurodegeneration in the brain, this can be permanent. But also, just like the brain this second brain has remarkable plasticity and it can relearn things and rewire itself, too.

The gut brain and our main brain are both loaded with thyroid hormone receptors. With Hashimoto's and hypothyroidism, there is often too little thyroid hormone or it's not getting absorbed properly.

This can result in damage to the enteric nervous system (the gut brain).

4. Problems with the Vagus nerve

The Vagus nerve is a central highway for communication between the brain and the gut. When the vagus nerve stops firing into the gut this slows down everything.

This is a major cause of slower motility and constipation.

344

Thyroid hormone has a direct affect on movement through the entire gastrointestinal tract.

Thyroid hormones increase intestinal neurotransmitters, increase blood flow to the intestines and support the repair and regeneration of the intestines.

Hypothyroidism can slow movement through the esophagus, can affect muscle function in this area and can affect the nerves that cause movement. Hypothyroidism also has an affect on the vagus nerve and this can lead both directly and indirectly to slowing movement through the intestines.

5. Anatomical or structural changes to the small intestines or illeosecal valve

Surgery to the gut (like appendectomy or resection), diverticulitis and scarring due to inflammatory bowel disease can all lead to this.

Hypothyroidism can lead to the loss of control of the ileosecal valve that is the doorway between the large and small intestine. When this stops working as it should it lets lots of critters from the large intestine into the small intestine.

Later in this chapter, we'll talk about testing and modifying the Autoimmune Diet for SIBO. Yeah. It's a project.

Recap

1. The small intestine is a busy place. Lots of nutrient absorption and sharing. Lots of immune cells and immune activity.

2. Consequently it's a place where a lot can happen, both good and bad. You can have an over active immune repines and flare ups.

You can have bacterial overgrowth and SIBO.

3. SIBO makes you a gas factory and can lead to lots of other issues, like digestive, skin related and neurological problems.

4. The answer is diet. Plain and simple.

HASHIMOMENT:
BE PRESENT & LISTEN TO YOUR HEART

In the West, your heart is associated with emotion. But in the Taoist tradition and in Chinese medicine, that is where you mind lives.

And many psychological disorders are treated as disturbances of shen or the spirit of the heart. These are treated using herbs and acupuncture that work on the heart and related channels.

What is also really interesting about this, is that if you have ever known anyone who has had a serous heart attack or open heart surgery, it is very common for that experience to radically transform their personality, really change them.

Of course, they come close to death, but also this has affected their hearts.

According to Taoist sage, Liu Yiming, "When the mind is open, it is aware; the original spirit is in charge of affairs, and illumination is managed properly. One can thereby balance yang.

When the mind is unruly, it wanders: the discriminatory consciousness handles affairs and illumination is not properly directed. This is sufficient to damage yang."

So what does this mean? Well, if you think about it, when we are aligned with our inner self, the heart and the mind function as one.

Following your heart is sometimes really difficult in the short term, but offers the biggest rewards in the long run. So the heart must rule and the mind must follow.

Sometimes easier said than done.

From the perspective of healing, only when our mind is able to spontaneously acknowledge and act on the truth within our hearts is healing complete.

It could be argued that connecting in this way to true self is to fulfill our individual destiny. This can take a life time.

The spirit of the heart, the shen, provides the means for us to reconnect to the true self stored in our depths. The heart rules the blood and the constancy of its beat reflects its commitment to fulfilling its role as sovereign ruler.

Hence a person's commitment may be seen as reflecting the quality of the heart's intention. One way to reunite the heart and mind is to think about your interpretation of the concept of commitment.

Meaning you should be to be 100% present while we are engaged in an activity.

One thing you can do to work on this is to be conscious of all the ways we avoid being present in daily life. Cell phones, tablets, TV, music, all conspiring to take us out of the present.

Meditation and morning prayer are good rituals to practice to get back in touch with our hearts.

Chapter Twenty-Seven

The Chinese Medicine View
of the Fire Element

Let's have a look at the Chinese medical take on the fire element.

Well, there are actually 4 body parts associated with the fire element. The heart and the pericardium are the yin organs. The heart is the actual organ, the pericardium is the protective membrane that surrounds the heart.

The yang organ is the small intestine and something unique to Chinese medical thought called the San Jiao. This is their way of talking about the pleural and peritoneal membranes that surround the lungs and the abdomen in the same way that the pericardium surrounds the heart.

These membranes hold many of the nerves and vessels supplying the organs of the abdomen and the lungs. Though the San Jiao is not recognized as an official organ in Western physiology, it does describe actual physiological functions and is important for water transfer and the function of digestive function.

Also, interestingly, in Chinese medicine, the heart is considered the master of the organ systems. It is the emperor.

The Nei Jing says "The heart holds the office of lord and sovereign. The radiance of the spirits stems from it."

Its sphere of influence includes: the vessels, the tongue, and it controls speech. Its negative emotion is joy (excessive or over-the-top joy) and its body fluid is sweat.

The heart's spirit is called the shen. Shen is like our soul, it's the spirit within us. It's what makes us unique and it is reflected in our mental, emotional and artistic expressions.

In the chapters on the Water Element, we discussed the concept of jing, which is the water in our well, our DNA, our potential energy. This is the yin aspect of our being.

Shen is jing's yang counterpart. It takes that potential energy and brings it into the world. It brings our latent abilities to life.

When the ancient Chinese spoke of the whole person, they referred to the shen-jing, the totality, the union of the spirit and the tangible parts of our life.

Our shen, or spirit, rises out of our jing (from our kidneys) and fills our hearts. Then this energy radiates out to all other organ systems. This forms a kind of heart/kidney axis.

This yin and yang energy of the jing and shen is expressed in all the organ systems of our bodies. And the shen is the yang part of this.

As we discussed, Hashimoto's involves a deficiency of yang and often our shen is tested mightily in this contest. An important manifestation of this energy is reflected in our commitment to things.

Healing Hashimoto's requires a strong sense of commitment. In order to be successful, we must keep trying and keep persevering in this contest. One thing that just breaks my heart is when I see people reach a point of hopelessness.

They know what they should be doing, but because they didn't get the results they hoped for they just say, "Screw it!" and return to eating whatever they want, ignoring the lifestyle changes that are so important.

This is another reason why the practices so beneficial for relieving stress, lowering reverse T3, and strengthening our shen are not luxuries or optional activities, in my opinion.

They are absolute necessities. We must cultivate this shen energy through meditation, prayer, affirmations or gratitude lists. Like any part of the body, this can be strengthened.

Another important ingredient to our success and something that can really help our commitment is a strong support network. Friends, family, and employers need to understand that we're in this for the long haul. And we must learn to communicate what we're going through.

Sometimes we can appear like we're doing fine on the outside, but on the inside we're falling apart. Another reason to cultivate shen energy is to give us the strength to ask for help.

In my experience, we can't do this alone. We need a strong support network of people who understand the magnitude of what we are trying to do.

The endocrine gland associated with the fire element is the pituitary. We've already seen how the pituitary is a master endocrine gland and how the Taoists believed that his is an important energy center.

So we can see that, on an energetic level, this is all connected as well. And that as we consciously work to strengthen these connections – to heal our brains, our kidneys and our hearts – we can make these connections begin to work for us and gather momentum in our healing process.

One small victory at a time.

Recap

Ok, so let's sum this up:

The spirit of the heart, the shen, provides the means for us to reconnect to the true self stored in our depths. The heart rules the blood and the constancy of its beat reflects its commitment to fulfilling its role as sovereign ruler.

Hence a person's commitment may be seen as reflecting the quality of the heart's intention. And it comes from our shen. We must cultivate this energy with exercises like meditation, qi gong, yoga.

Chapter Twenty-Eight

Other Parts of the Fire Element

Alright, now that your heart and mind have achieved oneness…

…let's look at the other parts of the fire element.

If the heart is the emperor or empress, the small intestine is the heart's closest minister and the go-between from the heart to the world and from the world into the heart.

Functionally, the small intestine helps us to clarify how we understand and express the truth and the spirit stored within our hearts and the hearts of others.

You don't usually get a private meeting with the emperor, more often it's his minister that first meets you to sort out what is important to convey to the heart.

And the opposite is also true; the top minister must also communicate the emperor's decisions to the outside world.

These basic principles are very much aligned with the actual functions of the small intestines.

It has to sort out what vitamins, minerals and amino acids, will be absorbed from food into the blood and delivered to the heart, and it must decide what waste is and what should be sent downward to the large intestine so it can be eliminated.

An important responsibility of the small intestine is to make sure that communication between the heart and mind, the heart and the outside world happens in a way that is aligned with virtue or integrity.

If the small intestine is not functioning properly, confusion can be the result. And we can misinterpret other's intentions and second guess ourselves.

The heart and the mind become separated and the heart can no longer communicate its insight.

Bitterness, the flavor associated with fire, may result from this misunderstanding.

Making unwanted advances or being sarcastic are examples of the small intestine being out of balance and not being able to convey's the heart's truth appropriately.

Listening is an important function of both the heart and the small intestine. People with small intestine imbalances may have difficulty listening to what you are saying.

The mind is so disconnected that what is being said and what occurs bear no relation to reality.

Or the person's interpretation of what is said is not at all what is being communicated. This can also manifest as a feeling of not being heard by others.

In a way, the small intestine focuses the intention of the heart. Balancing this relationship may be key to healing. This begins with learning how to listen. Meditation can develop this skill.

By becoming a better listener, you can better hear others and access your own inner truth.

The pericardium and the san jiao are also part of the fire element. They are unique in that they aren't really organs. They are really more like guards and protectors.

The pericardium according to the Nei Jing, "...has the charge of resident as well as envoy. Elation and joy stem from it."

Just as the emperor lived at the center of the forbidden city in ancient China, the heart lives at the center of the body surrounded by these other guards.

If the small intestine is the minister, the pericardium is like the guard who opens and closes the gate deciding who to let in and who to keep out.

Like a loyal body guard the pericardium receives the blows intended to strike the heart. Therefore, the pericardium plays a key role in many functional imbalances related to intimacy.

Using acupuncture on points of the pericardium channel can be very effective in helping to heal issues involving betrayal of intimacy.

According to the Nei Jing, the san jiao "....is responsible for opening up passages and irrigation. The regulation of fluids stems from it."

Physiologically the membranes of the san jiao help regulate water metabolism in the body. From an emotional point of view, the san jiao is like a customs guard at the border deciding who will be allowed to enter and leave the kingdom of the heart.

Remember the wei qi or defensive qi from the chapters on the Metal Element? The san jiao contributes to that. It keeps pathogens and emotional attackers outside and keeps them from entering the kingdom of one's heart.

Physiologically, the san jiao is also like the body's thermostat and it maintains balance by regulating fire (yang) and water (yin) throughout our bodies.

In order to do this, the san jiao has to maintain balance between the internal and external environments. It has to stay connected to our surroundings. In a way, it is responsible for gathering and sharing information the heart needs in order to rule effectively.

Healthy intimacy involves a balance between the pericardium and the san jiao. The virtue of the fire element is that it empowers maturity.

If the pericardium and san jioa are too strong, one may be overly protective of oneself and not allow intimacy.

If they are too weak and fire gets out of control one could be promiscuous and act out sexually, not caring about boundaries. Or this person can be an excessive talker who never let's anyone get a word in edgewise.

Treating acupuncture points on the san jiao channel can help regulate these boundaries. These are found along the ventral side of the forearm and on the upper back and head.

When the san jiao functions properly, we are not worried about establishing or avoiding connecting with others but simply acknowledging the nature of the connection that is already there.

Only by connecting to our own hearts and the hearts of others can we establish the alignment between heaven internally and externally that leads to fulfillment.

Ok, more insights, breakthroughs, hopefully no breakdowns, though sometimes breakdowns are part of this process. As we work on learning about and healing the fire element, we may be challenged.

And sometimes the biggest breakthroughs happen after the biggest breakdowns.

Recap

1. The fire element of Chinese medicine includes the heart, small intestine, pericardium and san jiao.

2. We saw how Hashimoto's and hypothyroidism can have a big impact on cardiovascular function and can really make you very

---

vulnerable to heart attack and stroke.

This makes what we learned earlier about blood sugar imbalances, metabolic syndrome and diabetes have special importance. You do not want to mess around here, people!

3. Emotionally and spiritually we looked at the fire element and the heart as the mind. Not the separation we see in the Western medical model, but something more unified.

A lot of this is about intimacy, and keeping the heart and the mind in alignment. Listening is really an important emotional and spiritual skill. It allows you to hear others and your own heart's direction.

Ultimately our goal is alignment with our true purpose and with heaven internally and externally.

The heart is the emperor or emperess and lives at the center of the body where it is protected by its loyal ministers and body guards.

You can do this. In my heart of hearts I know you can. All you need is some commitment and support. Together we can find hope, help, and healing by inspiring and supporting each other. At the very least, let's make a commitment to help each other.

Chapter Twenty-Nine

Using the A.P.A.R.T. System to Heal the Fire Element

A&A

T&T

P&P

R&R

A&A

The A.P.A.R.T. System

1. A = Ask and Assess

Your journal should be a book by now. Look for symptoms of problems with the Fire Element. Note what they are, then create a plan for addressing them. After that, you must act on your plan. Follow through and do what you have planned.

After that take inventory of what you did. Look at what worked and what didn't. Both will provide valuable information.

Double down on what worked, change what didn't. Summer is a good time to focus on healing fire elated issues. But, any time of year is a good time to heal the small intestines.

Heart Issues: Too much: Elevated heart rate, chest pain, high homocystein, high cholesterol, LDL, triglycerides, edema, high blood pressure

Too little: Slow heart rate, low blood pressure, anemia (see below for possible kinds)

Small Intestine Issues: Roughage and fiber cause constipation, Pain, tenderness, soreness on left side under rib cage, Stool undigested, foul smelling, mucous like, greasy or poorly formed, Frequent urination, Difficulty losing weight

Testing: Heart and Small Intestine

Ok, we've traveled pretty far down the fire road. Every time I look into something, lately, it seems to me that an entire universe of discovery awaits.

This is especially true with Hashimoto's. There is so much to learn, so much to explore, so much to discover.

And there are all these moving parts and connections.

I mean just look at this chapter, with the small intestine we really can see the convergence of the immune system, the cardiovascular system and the digestive system.

And everything is affecting everything else, either causing more vicious cycle downward spiral dominos or we start turning things around and we start to see all these connections working together to get us turned around and healed.

It's fascinating.

Ok, so in this last section today, I want to hit on some important things.

Firstly, I'd like to highlight 2 issues involving the blood that can torpedo your progress.

Earlier, we covered one of them, blood sugar imbalances. These must be dealt with and taken seriously and addressed or else you may really wind up in a world of hurt.

Because as we have seen, there are a whole boat load of additional cardiovascular risk factors added onto this equation by just simply being hypothyroid.

We saw seen how Hashimoto's and hypothyroidism can have a big impact on the heart and heart function.

And if you don't deal with your blood sugar issues, you can literally become a walking time bomb creating the perfect recipe for heart attack or stroke.

The second issue involving the blood is the various anemias. Anemias, like blood sugar imbalances can torpedo your progress and make all the time and money you are spending absolutely worthless.

Why? Because if you can't get enough oxygen and nutrients to your cells, they won't do you any good and you dramatically reduce your chances of recovering. You are always fighting a losing battle.

A Basic CBC: Complete Blood Count

You can get clues regarding anemias from a simple CBC, which costs about 15 bucks.

We looked at 3 anemias:

1. B12

2. Iron deficiency

3. Pernicious anemia

These can be seen in patterns of a basic CBC by looking at red blood cell counts and other related markers.

To learn more, visit the supplemental page on our website: https://hashimotos-diet.com/roadmap-to-remission-supplemental/

More on SIBO

The next thing that you may need to address is SIBO.

We talked about the main issues around SIBO, but wait there's more!

Many other symptoms of SIBO are a direct effect of nutrient malabsorption. This arises either from the bacteria metabolizing those nutrients before we can absorb them or by the bacteria causing enough inflammation in the lining of the gut that it the gut can't work properly anymore.

For example, the bacteria preferentially consume iron and vitamin B12, causing anemia. The bacteria decrease fat absorption by deconjugating bile leading to deficiencies of vitamins A & D and causing steatorrhea (fatty stools).

As the gut lining becomes increasingly inflamed and leaky, larger and not fully digested food particles enter the body, causing an immune reaction which leads to food allergies and food sensitivities.

Bacteria themselves can enter the blood stream causing systemic inflammation and immune reactions that can lead to autoantibody formation and autoimmune diseases.

There really is no end to these vicious cycles.

How Do You Test for SIBO?

In the conventional medical model there are 2 types of testing for SIBO. Both are flawed and not definitive.

1. Direct: Endoscopic Aspiration and Culture

This is a direct endoscopic aspiration and culture of the small intestine. This requires a gastroenterologist, it's expensive, it's invasive (they have to go in and get a sample).

The problem with this is that many of the bacteria removed from the small intestine can't be analyzed because they don't survive in culture.

Samples must be handled properly for accurate results.

To recap: It's expensive, it's invasive and sometimes tests don't reveal all the bacteria involved.

2. Indirect: Breath Testing for Hydrogen and Methane

This type of testing involves breath testing for hydrogen and methane.

This test can be inaccurate if someone has recently had antibiotics.

It may not be useful in determining all species of bacteria.
The optimal window for timing for collection is different for different people because transit time is different for different people.

To recap: You may get false negatives due to different transit times or antibiotic use.

Actually, the best test for SIBO is a trial diet and/or a stool test that looks for invasive species.

How Do you Fix SIBO?

Treatment Depends on Where You Are in the Progression

One important lesson that I have learned after working with over 1,000 people with Hashimoto's is that there are two really important things for getting good clinical results:

#1. Figure out the mechanism. In other words, where's the problem? With Hashimoto's it is often in multiple places and it's not only the thyroid.

#2. Figure out how advanced it is. Hashimoto's, like all autoimmune disease, is progressive. (Remember in the section on the Metal Element we discussed the 3 stages of progression.)

In a general sense, the further it has progressed the more you must do.

Healing By Subtraction

Another really valuable lesson I have learned is that, often, some of the most effective treatments and solutions come from subtraction.

Many common health problems are problems of excess. Too much sugar, too much stress, too much inflammation, too much salt, too many chemicals.

A simple and effective way of treating too much is by taking things away.
If you have insulin resistance or Type 2 diabetes, stop eating sugar and refined carbohydrates.

365

If stress is killing you, stop doing the things that cause you so much stress. If you have too much inflammation, stop eating and behaving in a way that causes so much inflammation.

If your sick from too much salt, stop eating salt.

If pollution is killing us and our world, stop using so many chemicals.

Such a simple solution, so hard to actually do.

At first.

The reason is that we are conditioned to be consumers, not subtractors.

However, if you have Hashimoto's, learning the habit of being content with less (sometimes a lot less) may just be the key to your healing.

Nowhere is this more true than in the treatment of SIBO

Diet Must Be the Foundation of Treatment

With SIBO, the foundation of treatment is diet because many of the bacteria feed on foods that are common in our diets.

And if you're like a lot of people I've worked with you might be asking yourself, "Why not just wipe them out with antibiotics?"

According to the American Journal of Gastroenterology, recurrence of small intestine bacteria after antibiotics is quite high (the most commonly prescribed being Rifaximin).

Many people have to keep taking antibiotics over and over again for months with limited results.

And there is a tremendous cost to your immune system and to your future ability to defend yourself.

(There is no better way to be defeated by an enemy than to give him repeated opportunities to adapt to your weapons.)

The only thing that really works is to do the diet as a foundation and then use something to eradicate the bacteria along with it.

There are a number of herbs that are quite effective for this. Particularly those in the berberine family like goldenseal, coptis, etc.

Probiotics Can Also Be Beneficial

A pilot study published in Acta Gastroenterologica Latinoamericana published in December 2010 found that probiotics may work better than pharmaceutical therapy for patients with chronic abdominal distention and SIBO.

"Based on this pilot study results, we can suggest that the probitoic herein (Lactobacillus casei, Lactobacillus plantarum, Streptococcus faecalis, Bifidobacterium brevis) used has a higher efficacy than metronidazonal in the early clinical response of patients with chronic abdominal distention and SIBO."

In the next section, we'll look into more treatment options for SIBO.

Recap

1. The fire element of Chinese medicine includes the heart, small intestine, pericardium and san jiao.

2. We saw how Hashimoto's and hypothyroidism can have a big impact on Cardiovascualr function and can really make you very vulnerable to heart attack and stroke.

This makes what we learned in Chapter 3 about blood sugar imbalances, metabolic syndrome and diabetes have special importance. You do not want to mess around here people!

3. Emotionally and spiritually we looked at the fire element and the heart as the mind. Not the separation we see in the Western medical model, but something more unified.

The heart is the emperor or emperess and lives at the center of the body where it is protected by its loyal ministers and body guards.

The fire element is all about relationships and learning to listen to our hearts so that we can become integrated internally and externally.

> **4. We looked at SIBO, another potential monkey wrench in the gears of our healing machine. It may take some time to fix this stuff people, be aware.**
>
> **Correcting SIBO can take up to 2 years. However, you should see improvement in your symptoms fairly quickly with gradual and continuous improvement.**

Stress, poor sleep, infections and poor diet choices can all create setbacks. It is always difficult to commit to more restrictive forms of a Paleo diet (which can be tough enough as it is!).

2. P = Prioritize and Plan

Not everything has the same level importance. This is what 80/20 teaches us. Some things are having more of an impact than others. Figure out which they are (the positive feedback loops) and then make a plan to fix them.

There's an awful lot here to evaluate. The small intestines, in my opinion, are ground zero for autoimmune disease and Hashimoto's. It could be argued that there is no other place more important to focus your treatment.

And because this is also where many important vitamins and minerals that are responsible for healthy thyroid function are absorbed this ecosystem must be kept healthy.

Finally, this is also where thyroid hormone is converted with the help of good bacteria.

The cardiovascular system is, of course, also important and if you have many of the risk factors mentioned in this section, I recommend focusing on the dietary elements that can heal the heart.

3. A = Act and Adapt

Act and put your plan into motion. Then observe what the results are. Double down on what works and change what doesn't. And results should be apparent relatively quickly. If they aren't you need to make changes.

Fire: Heart and Small Intestines

Foods:

Common Issues:

High Cholesterol: eat cholesterol lowering foods: apples, bananas, carrots, cold-water fish, garlic, grapefruit, olive oil, and fiber found in oats (gluten free). **Stop eating so much sugar:** Eliminate all refined sugars and flours.

Iron deficiency: dulse, kelp, rice bran, pumpkin seeds, beans, lentil, parsley, walnut, apricot, almond, raisins, swiss chard, spinach, dates, fig, kale, cucumber, cauliflower, cabbage

B12 deficiency: beef liver, beef kidney, ham, sole, scallops, eggs, oats, pickles, amasake, algae, spirulina and chlorella, brewer's yeast

B 6 deficiency: banana, barley, brewer's yeast, molasses, soybeans, wheat bran, brown rice, liver, beef, cabbage, carrots, potato, yams

High Homocysteine: Vitamin C, Vitamin E, Riboflavin, B6, Folate, B12 and magnesium are all helpful, the B vitamins especially.

-Dietary suggestions for calming and focusing the mind- Oyster shell, grain- brown rice, and oats, Mushrooms, Silicon foods- Oatstraw tea, oat groat tea, cucumber, celery, lettuce, Fruit- mulberries and lemons, Seeds-jujube seeds, Spices- dill and basil

Herbs/Supplements:
Dietary suggestions for calming and focusing the mind- chamomile, catnip, skullcap, valerian

Vitamins and Minerals:
B vitamins (See food sources in Chapter 1 for a complete list), Magnesium – found in chlorophyll foods, Amino acid L-tryptophan

The SIBO Diet

The SIBO diet is a terrific exercise in subtraction and should generally be done for a month or so to get the best results.

Since there are many foods that feed these bacteria, there are many foods that must be eliminated from your diet for this initial period of time.

Foods to Avoid:

Fructose: sugars, artificial sweeteners, corn syrup
Grains: rice, wheat, quinoa, millet, amaranth, and some non grains like tapioca
Legumes/Galactans: beans, peas, chickpeas, soybeans, lentils
Fructan-containing Vegetables: lettuce, onions, artichokes, beets, broccoli, cabbage, brussels sprouts, peas, asparagus, okra, shallots, mushrooms, green peppers, cauliflower
High-fructose fruits: grapes, apples, watermelon, cherries, kiwifruit, bananas, blueberries, mangos
Meat products: Breaded or processed meats such as hot dogs, bologna, potted meats, most cold cuts (added starches) and there are some who say to also avoid beef, pork and lamb.

Foods to Eat:

Nuts: All nuts except pistachios
Vegetables: All vegetables except those listed above
Low Fructose Fruits: apricots, avocados, cantaloupes, grapefruit, honeydew melons, nectarines, oranges, peaches, pineapples, raspberries, strawberries, tomatoes
Meats: chicken, fish, eggs, (and beef, lamb and pork in moderation)
Fats: Animal fat, oils

Steps of Treatment

The first step of treatment involves the diet as foundation and something to address the bacteria (like the herbs mentioned above).

Either during or after that Spartan menu, it is important to address the root causes and related issues of SIBO .

These problems include:

1. Too little stomach acid. Here's the exception to the healing by subtraction rule. If you have too little stomach acid, you need more.

A simple treatment is to take things that boost stomach acid levels such as apple cider vinegar, lemon juice and ginger root.

Supplementing with Betain HCL may also be beneficial (consult your doctor for this).

2. An immune suppressed gut. Often the cause of this is too much corticosteroid treatment and/or too much cortisol from stress.

Here the subtraction rule works quite well. Stop the corticosteroids (unless you have a condition where you must take them) and do something about stress.

A great daily exercise in doing less? Silent seated meditation.

3. Injury to the gut nervous system (The Enteric Nervous System)

This type of neurodegeneration is permanent. However, this nervous system also has remarkable plasticity and a capacity to rewire itself.

There are couple of really important things to do here:

#1. Vigorous, (I mean really vigorous to the point of tears) gargling. Gargle with several glasses of water throughout the day.

This activates part of the nervous system connected to the vagus nerve which has a very strong connection to the gut.

#2. Stimulate your gag reflex. Order some wooden tongue depressors online and gently stimulate this reflex by pressing down on the tongue.

#3. Coffee enemas. Make sure the coffee isn't too hot, and hold as long as possible. This causes nerve firing in the brain.

Start with a moderate amount and mild coffee, you can gradually increase both the amount of liquid and the strength of the coffee.

(Best to do it in the bathtub if you have one, so you are close to the toilet.)

How Long Do You Need to Treat SIBO?

Good question. You need to treat it for as long as it takes. And you may have to revisit this periodically. Generally speaking, the more severe it is, the longer and more committed you must be to healing it.

This may take several months.

It's also true that the better you are at really following the diet and not cheating, the better the outcome and the faster your results.

I and others like PaleoMom, Mickey Trescott, etc. recommend combining one of these diets with an Autoimmune Paleo diet for the most rapid and effective reversal of SIBO.

Recap

1. The fire element of Chinese medicine includes the heart, small intestine, pericardium and san jiao.

2. We saw how Hashimoto's and hypothyroidism can have a big impact on Cardiovascualr function and can really make you very vulnerable to heart attack and stroke.

This makes what we learned in Chapter 3 about blood sugar imbalances, metabolic syndrome and diabetes have special importance. You do not want to mess around here people!

3. Emotionally and spiritually we looked at the fire element and the heart as the mind. Not the separation we see in the Western medical model, but something more unified.

The heart is the emperor or emperess and lives at the center of the body where it is protected by its loyal ministers and body guards.

The fire element is all about relationships and learning to listen to our hearts so that we can become integrated internally and externally.

4. We looked at SIBO, another potential monkey wrench in the gears of our healing machine. It may take some time to fix this stuff people, be aware.

Correcting SIBO can take up to 2 years. However, you should see improvement in your symptoms fairly quickly with gradual and continuous improvement.

Stress, poor sleep, infections and poor diet choices can all create setbacks. It is always difficult to commit to more restrictive forms of a Paleo diet (which can be tough enough as it is!).

Qi Gong Exercise for the Fire Element

The Archer

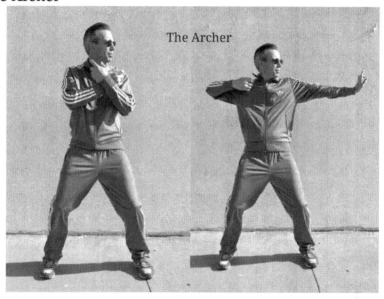

The Archer

In this exercise the opening and extending the chest and turning the head increases blood flow in your head, neck and chest area.It also improves heart and lung function. It's also a good excercise for improving posture and balance.

How to do it: Start in the Standing Form, feet shoulder width apart, weight evenly distributed. Bend your knees slightly. Use this same position for the entire exercise.

Next, inhale bring your arms in front of you chest in a crossed position about 6 inches in front of your heart with your palms facing towards your body and your right hand closer to your chest.

As you exhale, bring your gaze to your wrists. Focus on that spot, and in your mind, imagine that you are unstoppable. Next curl the fingers of your right hand as though you were drawing the string of a bow. Turn your left hand outward away from your body. Imagine you are drawing the bow with your right hand.

Next, inhale again and turn your head and use your eyes to follow your left arm all the way to your middle finger. Push away from your body with your left hand, extend your arm fully and point your palm straight up (at 90 degrees).

Imagine that your left hand is pushing a against something big like a mountain or a redwood. Atr the same time pull in the opposite direction with you right hand, until the right fist is even with the right shoulder.

And make sure the whole mobvement is slow and deliberate and not rushed.

Also, as you draw the bow, allow your hips to rotate toards your left hand a bit (this opens the lungs even more) and keep the knees bent. As the arms are fully stretched, focus on opening your chest, your lungs, your heart and your mind.

Finally exhale and return the hands to the crossed position in fron of your body. repeat the whole exercise in the opposite direction.

Repeat 3 times in both directions 1 or 2 times per day.

4. R= Reassess and Readjust

Retest, Reassess and ask all over again. Figure out what worked and what didn't. Double down on what worked and either eliminate or recreate a plan for what didn't.

With all the challenges that you may have to contend with in treating the Fire Element, it is very important to reassess and readjust.

Leaky gut, SIBO and other infections of the small intestines can be long term projects and it is not unusual for them to recur again in the future.
It's very much like growing a garden. A garden requires ongoing care. Planting, weeding, adding compost, harvesting, etc. The same is true of the ecosystem of the small intestines.

And the heart and related issues of the blood like anemias, and high cholesterol and homocysteine may need to rechecked periodically. And this has particular importance with Hashimoto's because of all the risk factors for heart attack and stroke.

5. T = Try and Try Again

Keep doing it, keep refining, keep building on the positive results and keep looking for the remaining positive feedback loops that are causing vicious cycles.

As I hope you have seen repeatedly throughout this book. The process of healing requires a long term commitment and an unwavering willingness to keep at it.

The larger goal of remission is the cumulative result of reaching many smaller goals first. It's important to acknowledge and celebrate these smaller victories, as well. They are the building blocks of success.

So pay attention, keep some kind of journal (physical or electronic) and keep building on what works and keeping evaluating and removing what doesn't serve your and your health.

In the final section of the book, I've created a "cheat sheet" that summarizes the most important areas (the 20%) that are priorities.

If you focus your attention on these areas, you will often find that you get results faster and that you can turn the tide against the downward spirals that can drag your mental, physical and emotional health downhill.

Put It Into Action

A Cheat Sheet for Finding Your 20%

HASHIMOTO'S HEALING CHEAT SHEET

In this final part of the book I'm going to break it all down for you. Everything you need to get started. And we'll look at in two ways: What you need to do and the mindset you need to have.

You can just skip to this section anytime you feel lost or need a reminder.

As I have shared in the introduction to this book, I believe in the 80/20 rule, that there's 20% of things that are causing 80% of your symptoms.

This Cheat Sheet covers the 20%.

Focus on these and, chances are, you'll see some improvement right away.

As you know, I've worked with an awful lot of people with Hashimoto's (this is all I do) and I've spent years studying and looking at research on how this condition impacts the body.

And the most important thing I have learned is that Hashimoto's is much more than a thyroid problem.

It's an autoimmune disease, but it's not just an immune system problem either. It's an all-over-your-body-problem.

Your body is not a machine. Like the earth, it's a complex group of ecosystems that all interact. And these ecosystems can all be adversely affected by Hashimoto's.

When this happens you get a downward spiral of vicious cycles all feeding on one another.

Positive Feedback Loops

This is caused by positive feedback loops, which is really just another way of saying things repeating over and over again with time.

These create webs that can lead to problems with virtually all the major systems of the body. These include issues with the brain, the adrenals, the liver and gall bladder and problems with the digestive tract like acid reflux, leaky gut, as well as body wide pain and inflammation and more.

And all of this can result in anxiety and depression, gall stones and poor liver detoxification, poor absorption of vitamins and nutrients, poor conversion of thyroid hormone, blood sugar imbalances, terrible fatigue and immune responses to various triggers from foods to environmental toxins and chemicals.

I admit I'm a bit obsessed with this, but there's an argument to made that problems every system you can imagine is caused by the ripple effect of hypothyroidism and autoimmunity on all the various systems of your body.

I've sometimes heard doctors shame their patients by saying, "People just try to blame everything on this disease." Well, that's because, everything is being caused by this disease. Thyroid hormone impacts virtually every system of the body.

So, it's not your fault.

However, now that you understand this, it's your responsibility to do something about it. You need to take your health into your own hands.

HOW DO YOU FIGURE OUT WHICH SYSTEMS ARE BREAKING DOWN?

This is half the battle. Once we answer this question, we can start fixing things.

First, you have to be able to see the big picture. Then identify which areas of your body need attention.

Create a plan for healing those areas and then execute that plan.

After you figure that out, you need to find the most destructive triggers and eliminate them. (The reality is that both of these things need to be done at the same time to get the best results.)

380

Where the Magic Happens

When you do these 2 things, something magical happens.

All of those vicious cycles get turned on their head and start having a positive impact on the other systems.

You start using positive feedback to your advantage. When that happens, you can stop triggering the immune system and start to restore balance.

Then the body can heal itself.

In the beginning, this will give you glimpses of more good days than bad ones and if you stay the course and work on the big picture you can even get this to remission.

(But remember that's not permission to go back to everything that got you sick in the first place.)

So, break that down into the changes you need to make.

STEP I: Start with the Diet

The diet is your foundation for healing. The gut is ground zero for autoimmunity and Hashimoto's. We have discussed this at length in this book.

In my experience, you're just spitting against Niagra Falls if you are trying to heal Hashimoto's without changing your diet.

The first thing you need to do is get started. Don't make excuses or rationalize why you're the exception. In most cases, you aren't the exception. Everyone with autoimmune disease has some degree of breakdown of their gut.

If you've been diagnosed with Hashimoto's, then you do too. So stop putting it off and stop waiting for the perfect time to get started. Now is the perfect time.

Test this approach first to determine whether or not it will benefit you. Don't decide before you tried it. And understand that this is a long term project. You might not get miraculous results right away.

If you're already on this diet and you aren't getting the results you had hope for. Check out this post in the supplemental section of our website on some of the potential reasons why: www.hashimtoshealing.com/r2rsupplemental

Get Your Mind Right:

Something else you need to come grips with is that this is a long term project. Like, really long. Basically, the rest of your life long.

Face it, accept it, and embrace the idea that from this point on, you're a "gut farmer" and weeding, cultivating, fertilizing, composting and healing the ecosystem of your gut is your vocation.

Get some cookbooks, start spending some time in the kitchen and the garden and get into it. It can be fun and incredibly rewarding if you just surrender and go for it.

What Diet Is Right For You?

I recommend starting with the strict Autoimmune Paleo diet, which means the elimination phase. You can ease into it and start by eliminating gluten, dairy and soy 100% or you can just jump into it and cut out everything.

Find a strategy that works for you. Get your family onboard and get some friends on board and support each other.

Once you get started, think of this diet as home base. Once you've gone through the intial elimination stage and slowly and carefully reintroduced things you may be able to venture off the farm every once in while, but don't go too far and always go back when you have a flare up of symptoms or start feeling crappy again.

And if you have gone too far, start all over again and go back to the elimination diet 100%.

Now, this diet is the foundation and it is home base, but it may not solve all your problems. And you may need to tweak it for your particular set of circumstances.

Some people do better with a bit more carbohydrates and adding more resistant starches may be be something you need to do.

But, first, you need to start, you need to get some data from the experience of doing it and then you need analyze and reassess (use the A.P.A.R.T. system) and make changes and adjustments as necessary.

STEP 2: Start Investigating the Other Systems of Your Body and Start Putting Together Your Healing Action Plan

Let's review those:

I. Your Brain : (Let's start at the top and work our way down. :))

Many of the most common symptoms of Hashimoto's are brain based.

Meaning they come from the brain.

For example, fatigue, brain fog and memory issues, depression, anxiety, constipation and more can all come from how the brain is affected by hypothyroidism and autoimmunity.

To learn more about this, check out this video series:

SAVE YOUR BRAIN (FROM HASHIMOTO'S):
https://www.hashimotoshealing.com/savingbrain/

Here's a few things that a healthy Hashimoto's brain needs (and, as it turns out, all of these things are also beneficial to your thyroid and the rest of your body):

1. Sugar: The brain is the body's biggest consumer of sugar

However, this is not a license to hammer Snickers bars.

The key is to not have too much or too little. There's a "Goldilocks" zone. If you're hypoglycemic, make sure your sugar doesn't crash. (See below for a more in depth discussion)

If you're a sugar addict, admit it, stop living in denial and get help. Treat your addiction.

2. Oxygen: The brain needs oxygen

Iron deficiency and other anemia can put a hurt on your brain. Don't do that. Get an iron panel, and check your ferritin. Order a CBC and check red blood cell values. Check hemoglobin, RBC and other red blood cell values.

3. Blood flow: The brain needs blood flow.

Many people with Hashimoto's and hypothyroidism have low normal blood pressure. That's not always a good thing. Low blood pressure is a major risk factor for Alzheimer's. So get blood flowing to your brain.

If your blood pressure is consistently low try adding some salt, especially sea salt or Himalyan salt as they are high in trace minerals.

Also, anemia is a big problem for the brain. You can't be even a little iron deficient or B12 deficient or any other kind of deficient.

Rule these things out. If you have them, they must be dealt with. Being even "a little anemic" is big deal. It has major consequences.

4. Less Inflammation: Inflammation is the root of all evil.

An inflamed brain is not a good thing. Just ask former NFL players.

Inflammation of any kind in the brain can take a long time to resolve. When you have brain inflammation, the immune system in the brain goes into overdrive and starts destroying brain cells in the process.

No bueno.

Try turmeric and lots of it.

5. Sleep: So important, yet so overlooked.

Turn off the tv. Move it out of the bedroom if you need to. Think of sleep as the most important thing you can do for you health. If you're having trouble sleeping, read on.

Get Your Mind Right: Brain inflammation is no joke. This can progress to Alzheimer's or Parkinson's-like symptoms. Hashimoto's can lead to major degeneration of your brain.

It's not your fault, but it is your responsibility to do something about it.

Since the gut and the brain are so closely related, you kind of need to be a brain framer as well as a gut farmer. And, the good news is, healthy choices in one area benefits the other.

II. Endocrine Land: The Adrenals & The Pancreas: (Moving from the Brain to the Endocrine glands)

For a lot of people with Hashimoto's the adrenals are a critical piece of the puzzle.

The warning the label on Synthroid and other thyroid replacement hormone warns that if a patient has adrenal insufficiency they should not be prescribed the drug?

That's how important the adrenals are.

They can be the difference between you turning this thing around and you treading water and not improving or just continuing to get worse.

In our practice we do proper testing evaluation and treatment of the adrenals. The best test is the ASI or Adrenal Salivary Index. I also gave you some other tests in the Chapters on the Water Element.

And, of course, it does no good to just test and not do anything about stress. For the vast majority of us Hashimoto's folks, stress can cause major problems.

You don't need testing to understand this.

When you are stressed, you can have more immune flare ups and this can trigger your Hashimoto's and make it worse.

So, what are doing about stress?

You need to actually be doing things. Meditating, resting, getting massages, doing yoga and/or qi gong, going for walks in Nature, having fun.

This is not optional or some luxury that you treat yourself with once a year. This needs to be a daily part of your regimen.

Because, here's the tricky thing about adrenal stress: it's almost always caused – at least in part – by something else.

These causes include anemia, blood sugar swings, gut inflammation, food intolerances (especially gluten, dairy and soy), essential fatty acid deficiencies, environmental toxins, and of course, chronic emotional and psychological stress.

Sound familiar?

These are also all the things that make Hashimoto's worse.

We can't ignore them or pretend like they aren't there. We have to deal with all of them.

We have maxed out our stress cards (like our credit cards for stress). With Hashimoto's your body is under so much physiological stress, all the time, that extra emotional stress will often totally wipe you out.

This happens because we've emptied our accounts and now we have to start putting relaxation and fun back into our "stress savings" accounts.

Seriously, you have to replenish this account. It's not enough to say "Yeah, I have nothing in that account."

Because just like your bank account if you aren't putting money back in and you're always just taking money out, what happens?

Eventually, you go broke and you got all these creditors after you and lose your house and your car and eventually, you wind up on the street.

Talked about stressed out!

That's what's happening in your body. You wind up with the functional equivalent of being homeless inside your own body.

So, come up with an actual stress strategy. This means real action items, things that you are going to do on a daily, weekly and monthly basis for yourself to stop stress from preventing you from getting any better.

III. Blood Sugar Problems

Welcome to the Blood Sugar Vicious Cycle

Both high blood sugar and low blood sugar levels can make your Hashimoto's worse.

These spikes and crashes of blood sugar adds significant stress to the body, cauases your adrenals to pump out cortisol which makes the gut breakdown, makes thyroid hormone not work as well and pushes autoimmunity.

You have to deal with sugar like it's one of your top priority issues.

If you are hypoglycemic, you can't let your blood sugar crash, you must be on top of this and make sure you always have something to snack on and that you do not allow yourself to get to irritable, angry, spacey, forgetful or really hungry.

If you reach that point, it's too late.

Instead, start the day with a good protein and fat combination, eat every few hours, and avoid high sugar foods and refined carbohydrates that will make you spike and crash to the floor like a lead balloon.

If you are insulin resistant and/or you've been diagnosed with metabolic syndrome or Type II diabetes, then chances are you are a sugar addict.

Sugar is more addictive and, arguably, more dangerous than cocaine for people with Hashimoto's. You have to treat it as such.

If you follow the Autoimmune Paleo diet to the letter, it will help. But you may need to do a sugar detox and really go cold turkey and see just how bad it is.

Get Your Mind Right: Sugar is not your friend. It's not a good source of energy, it may provide some comfort, but that comfort is short lived and it comes with a nice helping of increased suffering.

Let go of sugar, set yourself free. Look for other ways to get a rush of dopamine into your life.

Like exercise, meditation, qi gong, yoga, walking in Nature, sex and intimacy, art and music. There are other ways to feel good.

It's Another Vicious Cycle

If you want to heal your Hashimoto's, you need to deal with blood sugar issues. And that means dealing with your sugar habit.

IIV. Last but Definitely Not Least: Heal Your Gut

The more I study and learn, the more research I see and the more people I work with I am convinced that the gut is ground zero for autoimmunity. It's a place of maximum leverage.

It may be in the top 5-10% of the 20%.

Investing in healing the gut is an investment that can give you a three to ten times return on your investment.

It's worth every bit of time, energy, effort and money you put into it.

And real gut health begins with what you put in your mouth and then continues on down your digestive tract.

I'm always shocked when patient tell me their doctors say, "Diet doesn't matter."

This reflects an extraordinary level of ignorance. It's a lie and ignoring this leads a lot of people to get a lot sicker.

Here's a post that discusses this and gives you a good perspective on a diet for Hashimoto's.

Hashimoto's Diet: Keys to Success
https://hashimotos-diet.com/roadmap-to-remission-supplemental/

In addition, many doctors also say going gluten free is a fad and isn't such a big deal.

This is also absurd when you look at the research.

Here's another post in which we have done just that, tons of it:

Gluten, Celiac Disease and Hashimoto's
https://hashimotos-diet.com/roadmap-to-remission-supplemental/

And every organ along the way needs to be examined and healed, if necessary.

This begins with the stomach.

Hashimoto's and hypothyroidism can cause too little stomach acid to be secreted which leads to problems all down the line.

So, start with your stomach.

Review the Earth Element section on stomach acid issues.

Once you've addressed the stomach, you need to make sure the pancreas is functioning properly and we have discussed that in detail already.

Balance your blood sugar.

From there it's the liver and gall bladder.

These are also hugely important.

Review the chapters on the Wood Element.

From there we move onto the real home of autoimmune disease, the small intestines.

This is where it all began and where it continues to flourish if you don't do something about it.

One big issue we discussed at length is leaky gut.

Heal the environment of the intestines. Understand that parasites, yeast, and bacterial overgrowth can all be potential problems.

Guess what often helps all of those? Cutting out all refined sugars.

Another complication we find is something called SIBO which stands for Small Intestine Bacterial Overgrowth.

This can be caused by too little stomach acid and can lead to leaky gut and all of these things can make each other worse.

You'll find links to a 2 part series I wrote that goes into depth on SIBO here: https://hashimotos-diet.com/roadmap-to-remission-supplemental/

And there you have it.

A quick overview of the most common issues that need fixing.

Get to work on those areas and, chances are, you'll start to feel a whole lot better.

Get Your Mind Right: Your gut is ground zero. Your health and recovery depends on it getting healed. Invest in gut healing.

Become a gut farmer. Make this your vocation, your passion, your expertise.

Heal the Earth Element. While we're at it, let's heal the planet Earth too.

You Aren't Alone

Well, you aren't alone in this.

And you aren't going to fix everything in a day or 2.

First step is to identify where the problems are.

The next step is to figure which systems are in the worst shape and start with healing those.

Then you need to keep moving onto the other systems and periodically circle back to the big ones and reevaluate.

It's not as hard as it seems.

It just takes a little commitment and focus.

And it really helps to have a plan.

If you want help, I'm here for you.

Join me on the Road to Remission.

If you want to talk to me and learn more, you can also contact me at marc@hashimotoshealing.com and/or set up a free 30 minute Hashimoto's Healing Discovery Session.

In it you can share where you are and where you want to be, I can make some recommendations right away and we can discuss how working together can get you better faster.

Here's a link to set up a time to chat. (Fair warning, these are booked out at least 2 to 3 months in advance.)

Schedule a Free 30 Minute Session with Marc
If you want to get started sooner, just send me an email and let me know and I'll open up a time for you before then.

Finally, here's a reminder of the A.P.A.R.T. System that is designed to take the guess work out of this process and is guaranteed to keep you on track and to get results if you use it.

The A.P.A.R.T. System

A&A

T&T

P&P

R&R

A&A

The A.P.A.R.T. System

Apply the A.P.A.R.T. System to all top areas we just mentioned in the Cheat Sheet.

1. Your Brain

2. Your Adrenals

3. Blood Sugar Imbalances

4. Your Gut

5. Your Stomach

6. Your Liver

7. Your Intestines

    1.   A = Ask and Asses

Data has healing power, if you know what data to collect and analyze and you know what to do with that information. (Both are big "if"'s).

You need to ask what the symptoms are and assess the different systems of the body to find out where these symptoms are coming from.

And everything needs to be a suspect. Don't exclude something because you're attached to it or feel like you can't do without it. Everything in your life should be evaluated and if it isn't working to make you better, it should be eliminated.

This includes people, places and things like your favorite foods and drinks.

2. P = Prioritize and Plan

Not everything has the same level importance. This is what 80/20 teaches us. Some things are having more of an impact than others. Figure out which they are (the positive feedback loops), focus on those first and then make a plan to fix them.

Use the Cheat Sheet to identify the top suspects that are causing 80% of your problems.

3. A = Act and Adapt

Act and put a plan into motion.

Use the foods and Qi gong exercises from this book and incorporate them into your life every day.

Then observe what the results are. Double down on what works and change what doesn't. And results should be apparent relatively quickly. If they aren't you need to make changes.

The common practice of prescribing something and then telling the patient to come back in 3 to 6 months is ridiculous, in my opinion. That's way too long, especially if it isn't working.

4. R= Reassess and Readjust

Retest, Reassess and ask all over again. Figure out what worked and what didn't. Double down on what worked and either eliminate or re-create a plan for what didn't.

It sounds obvious, but it is often overlooked or forgotten. Testing and re-evaluating what you have done to see the result of your treatment is essential for good care.

Quick side note here: In my opinion, what I have learned over many years of practice is that you need to trust what the data is telling you. In most cases, when you make the right choice you start feeling better.

Things like a "healing crisis", a "die off" or a "detox reaction" sometimes occur, but they can also be a cover for incompetence. The right decision should result in a positive result relatively quickly.

If you are doing something and you aren't getting better or you continue to feel worse or it causes more discomfort, pain and adverse symptoms then you need to question whether or not that is the best course of action.

Eliminate it, reduce variables and find out which part of what you are doing is causing that reaction or set of symptoms.

And all of this should not be done on the basis of lab tests alone. With Hashimoto's it must include a thorough examination of the signs and symptoms as well.

Remember, what you feel is diagnostically important and clinically relevant.

5. T = Try and Try Again

Keep doing it, keep refining, keep building on the positive results and keep looking for the remaining positive feedback loops that are causing vicious cycles.

People sometimes give up before giving a certain approach a chance. Or they get some good results and then slide back to their old ways of doing things. When you find something that works, keep doing it. Don't quit and don't give up.

Success is defined by the transformation of a vicious cycle into positive healing momentum. This means you start to feel better and then exponentially better.

Lab work and symptoms should all confirm that this has taken place.

You can do this!

If you need help, you know where to find me:
marc@hashimotoshealing.com

Yours in Remission,
Marc Ryan, L.Ac.

References & Notes:

Preface:

After creating the A.P.A.R.T. System, I discovered "biohacking" and noticed some similarities. The main point is that we need an approach that is adaptable to change and that provides us with a blueprint for long term improvement. The current Western medical model doesn't empower the patient with tools for adaptation and progressive improvement, in my opinion.

Introduction:

"Synthroid Sales Data." Drugs.com. Drugs.com, 1 Feb. 2014.

"The hypothyroid medication levothyroxine (*Synthroid*, AbbVie) continues to be the nation's most prescribed drug"

"The Best Clinical Guidelines Money Can Buy: A look at Guidelines Bias and Thyroid Treatment." *Holtorf Med*. Holtorf Medical Group.

"The American Association of Clinical Endocrinologists (AACE) and the American Thyroid Association (ATA) put together a task force on adult hypothyroidism, and published their "Clinical Practice Guidelines for Hypothyroidism in Adults (The "Guidelines") in 2012.

The result was jointly published in 2012 in the journals *Thyroid* and *Endocrine Practice*.

According to the authors, the Guidelines present "evidence-based recommendations" that, according to the report, "were developed to aid in the care of patients with hypothyroidism and to share what the authors believe is current, rational and optimal medical practice for the diagnosis and care of hypothyroidism."

The authors included Jeffrey R. Garber, Rhoda H. Cobin, Hossein Gharib, James V. Hennessey, Irwin Klein, Jeffrey I. Mechanick, Rachel Pessah-Pollack, Peter A. Singer, and Kenneth A. Woeber. In the published guidelines' reference to financial disclosures, only Jeffrey

Mechanick was listed as having any financial ties, in this case to Abbott, parent company of AbbVie, which manufactures Synthroid.

While the other guidelines committee members claimed they had "no relevant financial relationships with any commercial interests," this is not true. A search of the ProPublica "Dollars for Doctors" database shows that committee member Rhoda Cobin has financial ties to drug companies.

Peter Singer has disclosed in other venues that he is a consultant for Abbvie Pharmaceuticals, maker of Synthroid. Hossein Gharib and James Hennessey have also been speakers at AbbVie financed symposia.

Not only do many of the guidelines committee members have clear ties to the drug industry, and in particular, the company that makes the top-selling brand of levothyroxine, but the guidelines' disclosures were less than forthcoming.

AbbVie, a spinoff of Abbott Labs, is the key player in the levothyroxine market, as it manufactures thyroid drug Synthroid, the top-selling brand name of levothyroxine. AbbVie spreads around millions of dollars a year financing workshops, symposia, training sessions, and other industry events, and providing direct support to many physicians in the form of honoraria, speaker's fees, drug samples, and other payments.

Levoxyl, owned by pharma powerhouse Pfizer, is a secondary, but important player. In contrast, the makers of T3 and natural thyroid drugs have limited marketing budgets, face heavy regulations on what sort of marketing they can do (especially for regulatory-grandfathered natural thyroid drugs), and are not typically involved in financing thyroid and endocrinology guidelines members or their organizations.

So did the industry ties of the committee members, and the influence of the levothyroxine manufacturer, show up in the Hypothyroidism Guidelines?

Take a look at the following recommendations from the Guidelines:

- Patients with hypothyroidism should be treated only with levothyroxine drugs.

- The evidence does not support using levothyroxine-plus-T3 combinations to treat hypothyroidism.

- There is no evidence to support using natural desiccated thyroid hormone — i.e., Armour, Nature-Throid — in preference to levothyroxine in treating hypothyroidism. The Guidelines conclude that "therefore desiccated thyroid hormone should not be used for the treatment of hypothyroidism.

The Guidelines also include the following statements:

- Thyroid Stimulating Hormone (TSH) is the single best screening test for primary thyroid dysfunction for the vast majority of outpatient clinical situations.

- The standard treatment is replacement with levothyroxine (T4).

- The decision to treat subclinical hypothyroidism, when the serum TSH is less than 10 mIU/L, should be tailored to the individual patient."

At the time of writing this book I have had 2325 consultations with Hashimoto's patients. I had 1093 free consultations and 432 clients. I have tallied more detailed data on the clients but we are still studying this data.

I surveyed 904 individuals who were diagnosed with Hashimoto's. These took place from April 2013 to June 2015. The average age was 46, 870 were female, 34 were male. 502 were on thyroid replacement hormone, 402 were not. The most commonly prescribed was Synthroid, followed by Levothyroxine, Armour and Naturethroid. Most common symptoms included fatigue, brain fog, weight gain, depression, anxiety, hair loss/thinning hair, constipation and insomnia.

Muchof what I have observed in clinical practice and in these conversations is shared in this book.

Ho TW et al. Utilization of Thyroidectomy for benign disease in the United States: a 15-year population based study. Am J Surg

2011:201:570-4

Summary of the Study

"The authors found that the percentage of patients having total thyroidectomy increased from 17.6% (from 1993-1997) to 39.4% (from 2003-2007) for benign, non-cancerous, thyroid disease.

While there was very little variation across different regions of the United States, patients were most likely to undergo total thyroidectomy at an urban teaching hospital than in urban non-teaching or rural hospitals.

The Authors also found that the length of time spent in the hospital and the hospital charges were significantly more for total thyroidectomy. The data also demonstrated a higher rate of post-operative complications with total thyroidectomy, such as low calcium levels, bleeding and hoarseness due to vocal cord problems.

Hospitals that performed a higher number of thyroid operations were found to have lower complication rates."

Azad, Kalid. "Understanding the Pareto Principle (The 80/20 Rule)." *Better Explained.*

Chapter 1: Functional Medicine and the 5 Elements of Thyroid health

Ni, Hua-Ching. Tao, The Subtle Universal Law and the Integral Way of Life. Tao of Wellness, Santa Monica. Ca. 2014.

Beinfield, Harriet, Korngold Efrem. Between Heaven and Earth. Ballantine, 1991.

Wilder, G.D, Ingram J.H. Analysis of Chinese Characters.
New York: Dover Publications, 1974.

Kaptchuk, Ted J. The Web That Has No Weaver: Understanding Chinese Medicine. Congdon and Weed, Inc.1983.

Descotes J, Vial T. Immunetoxic effects of xenobiotics in humans: A review of current evidence. *Toxicol in Vitro*.1994 Oct;8(5):963-966

Steventon GB, heafield MT, Sturman S, Waring RH, Williams AC. Xeno biotic metabolism in Alzheimer's disease. *Neurology*. 1990;40:1095-1098.

Ridgen S. Evaluation of the effect of modified entero-hepatic resuscitation program in chronic fatigue syndrome patients. *J Adv Med*. 1998;11(4):247-262

Mckinnon RA. Possible role of cytochromes P450 in lupus erythematosus and related disorders. *Lupus*.1994;3:473-478

Braverman, Lewis E., and Robert D. Utiger. "Section C. Organ System Manifestations of Hypothyroidism." Werner & Ingbar's-The Thyroid: A Fundamental and Clinical Text. 9th ed. Philadelphia: Lippincott Williams & Wilkins, 2005. 769-850.

2-5: (Thyroid)

Gibson, Peter R., and Susan J. Shepherd. "Evidence Based Dietary Management of Functional Gastrointestinal Symptoms: The FODMAP Approach." Journal of Gastroenterology and Hepatology (2010): 252-58.

Kharrazian, Datis. Mastering Functional Blood Chemisry. Datis Kharrazian, 2012.

Laboratory Evaluations for Integrative and Functional Medicine, 2nd Edition, Richard S. Lord, J. Alexander Bralley, 2008

Kharrazian, Datis. Mastering the Thyroid. Datis Kharrazian, 2011.

Braverman, Lewis E., Utiger, Robert D. "Part II Laboratory Assessment of Thyroid Function.", "Section B-Causes of Hypothyroidism" Werner & Ingbar's-The Thyroid: A Fundamental and Clinical Text. 9th ed. Philadelphia: Lippincott Williams & Wilkins, 2005. 309-373,701-714.

Flaws, Bob, Sionneau Philippe. "Hashimoto's Thyroiditis." The Treatment of Modern Western Medical Diseases with Chinese Medicine: A Textbook and Clinical Manual. Boulder: Blue Poppy, 2001. 241-246.

Kendall, Donald E. Dao of Chinese Medicine: Understanding an Ancient Healing Art. Oxford: Oxford UP, 2002.

Lakatos P., Thyroid hormones: beneficial or deleterious for bone? Calcif Tissue Int. 2003. Sep;73(3):205-9

Muller MJ, Burger AC, Ferrannini E, et al. Glucoregulatory function of thyroid hormones; role of pancreatic hormones. Am J Physio. 1989;256:E101-E110

Calza L, et al. Thyroid hormone-induced plasticity in the adult rat brain. Brain Res Bull. 1997;44(4):549-57

Flavin RSL, et al. Regulation of microglial development: a novel role for thyroid hormones. The Journal of Neuroscience. 2001;21(6):2028-2038Oge

A, Sozmen E, Karaoglue AO. (2004) Effect of thyroid function on LDL oxidation in hypothyroidsim and hyperthyroidism. Endocr Res 2004; 30:481-489

Laukkarinen J, Kiudelis G, Lempinen M, Raty S, Pelli H, Sand J, Kemppainen E, Haglund C, Nordback I. Increased prevalence of subclinical hypothyroidism in common bile duct stone patients. J Clin Endocrinol Metab. 2007 Nov;92(11):4260-4.

Epub 2007 Aug 28Inkinen J, Sand J, Nordback I. Association between common bile duct stones and treated hypothyroidism. Hepatogastroenterology. 2000 Jul-Aug:47(34):919-21

Napoli R, Guarasole V, Angelini V, et al. Acute effects of triiodothyronine on endothethial function in human subjects. J Clin Endocrinol Metabl. 2007;92(1):250-4

Taddei S, Caraccio N, Virdis A, et al. Impaired endothelium-dependent vasodilation in subclinical hypothyroidism: beneficial effect of levothyroxine therapy. J Clin Endocrinal Metab. 2003:88(8):2731-7

Pustorino S., Foti M., Calipari G., Pusterino E., Ferrero R., Guerrisi O., Germanotta G., Thyroid-intestinal motility interactions summary. Minerva Gastroenterol Dietol. 2004 Dec;50(4):305-15

Green JR, Diminished TSH repines to TRH stimulation in patients with hepatic cirrhosis dispute subnormal T3 levels. Z. Gastroenterol. 1979:17(7):447-51

Saha B, Maity C. Alteration of serum enzymes in primary hypothyroidism. Clin Chem Lab Med. 2002;40:609-611Purandare A, Godil M, Ahnn SH, et al. Effect of hypothyroidism and its treatment on IGF system in infants and children, J Pediatr Endocrinol metal. 2003;16:35-42

The Journal of Clinical Endocrinology & Metabolism 2005; 90(12):6403–6409

Depression and hypothyroidism:

This is an area of considerable controversy because these drugs are sometimes prescribed without a proper work up of the thyroid and these medications have been shown to impact iodine availability, affect peroxidase activity and stimulate conversion.

Jarrett, Lonny S. "The Five Elements." Nourishing Destiny: The Inner Tradition of Chinese Medicine. Stockbridge: Spirit Path, 1998. 121-136.

Thyroid Hormone Concentrations, Disease, Physical Function and Mortality in Elderly Men Annewieke W. van den Beld, Theo J. Visser, Richard A. Feelders, Diederick E. Grobbee, and Steven W. J. Lamberts Department of Internal Medicine

RR, Scobbo. et al"Serum TSH Variability in Normal Individuals: The Influence of Time of Sample Collection." W V Med J. 2004 Jul-Aug;100(4):138-42

Brown, Judith. "Food Sources of Vitamins and Minerals." *Epi.umn.edu.* University of Minnesota, Division of Epidemiology.

Virion, A., et al., "Opposite Effects of Thiocyanate on Tyrosine Iodination and Thyroid Hormone Synthesis", Eur J Biochem. 1980;112(1):1-7

Yuan, G. J., et al., "Effects of Different Cooking Methods on Health-Promoting Compounds of Broccoli". J Zhejiang Unvi Sci B. 2009;10(8):580-588

Zimmermann. M. B. and Kohrle, J., "The Impact of Iron and Selenium Deficiencies on Iodine and Thyroid Metabolism: Biochemistry and Relevance to Public Health", Thyroid. 2002;12(10):867-78

Lee, Ju-Han et al. "The Association between Papillary Thyroid Carcinoma and Histologically Proven Hashimoto's Thyroiditis: A Meta-analysis." Eje-online.org. European Society of Endocrinology, 2012.

Trentini, Dana. "Top 5 Reasons Doctors Fail To Diagnose Hypothyroidism." *Hypothyroid Mom.* Prose Theme on Genesis Framework, 26 Nov. 2012.

"Rt3-ratio." *Stop the Thyroid Madness.* Stop the Thyroid Madness.

"Thyroid Hormone Transport." *Nahypothyroidism.* National Academy of Hypothyroidism.

What about Goitrogens in Cruciferous Vegetables?
Ballantyne, Sarah. "The Paleo Approach Diet." *The Paleo Approach: Reverse Autoimmune Disease and Heal Your Body.* Victory Belt, 2013. 209-210.

Clinical Manual of Oriental Medicine: An Integrated Approach. 2nd ed. Industry: Lotus Institute of Integrative Medicine. Print.

Chapter 6-9 (The Metal Element):

Kern, S., and T. Ziemssen. "Psychoneuroimmunology--cross-talk between the Immune and Nervous Systems." *Ncbi.nlm.nih.gov.* J Neurol. 2007 May;254 Suppl 2:II8-11.

Yaghini, N. et al."Serum Levels of Interleukin 10 (IL-10) in Patients with Type 2 Diabetes." Iran Red Crescent Med Jv.13(10);2011.Oct

Chen, John K., Chen, Tina T. Chinese Medical Herbology and Pharmacology. Industry: Art of Medicine, 2001.

Corthay, A. "How Do Regulatory T Cells Work?" Scand J Immunol. 2009 Oct; 70(4): 326–336.

Kendall, Donald E. Dao of Chinese Medicine: Understanding an Ancient Healing Art. Oxford: Oxford UP, 2002.

Jarrett, Lonny S. "Metal-The Return." Nourishing Destiny: The Inner Tradition of Chinese Medicine. Stockbridge: Spirit Path, 1998. 258-276.

Th1/Th2 Balance: The Hypothesis, its Limitations, and Implications for Health and Disease, Parris Kidd, PhD Alternative Medicine Review, Volume 8, Number 3 2003

Kharrazian, Datis. Mastering the Thyroid. Datis Kharrazian, 2011.
Kharrazian, Datis. Why Do I Still Have Thyroid Symptoms?:When My Lab Tests Are Normal. Carlsbad: Elephant Printing, LLC, 2010.

Benschoten, Van. Autoimmune Disease and Chinese Herbal Medicine. Santa Monica. Ca: Emperor's College of Oriental Medicine, 2003.

Autoimmune Disease, Multiple Chemical Disorders, and Chinese Medicine, M.M. Van Benchotten, O.M.D., Lotus Institute of integrative Medicine, 2009

The Immune Response: Basic and Clinical Principles By Tak W. Mak, Mary E. Saunders, Academic Press, 2005 page 451-3

"Autoimmune Statistics." *Aarda.org*. American Autoimmune Related Diseases Association, Inc.

Trentini, Dana. "Hashimoto's: Your Body Is Not Supposed To Destroy Itself Right?" *Hypothyroid Mom*. Prose Theme on Genesis Framework, 3 Dec. 2012.

DY, Aksoy et al. "Effects of Prophylactic Thyroid Hormone Replacement in Euthyroid Hashimoto's Thyroiditis." Endocr J. 2005 Jun;52(3):337-43

Kresser, Chris. "Basics of Immune Balancing for Hashimoto's." *ChrisKresser.com*. Chris Kresser, 30 Aug. 2010.

"Nitric Oxide Modulation for Autoimmune Disease." *Drknews.com* Datis Kharrazian, 13 Mar. 2012.

Drugarin D. The pattern of Th1 cytokine in autoimmune thyroiditis. Immunol Letts, 2000; 71: 73-77

McGrogan A, Seaman HE, Wright JW, de Vries CS. The incidence of autoimmune thyroid disease: a systematic review of the literature. Clin Endocrinol (Oxf). 2008 Nov;69(5):687-96. doi: 10.1111/j.1365-2265.2008.03338.x. Epub 2008 Jul 31.

Boelaert K, Newby PR, Simmonds MJ, Holder RL, Carr-Smith JD, Heward JM, Manji N, Allahabadia A, Armitage M, Chatterjee KV, Lazarus JH, Pearce SH,Vaidya B, Gough SC, Franklyn JA.
Prevalence and relative risk of other autoimmune diseases in subjects with autoimmune thyroid disease. Am J Med. 2010 Feb;123(2):183.e1-9. doi: 10.1016/j.amjmed.2009.06.030.

"What Is Celiac Disease?" *Csaceliacs.org*. Celiac Support Association/United States of America, Inc.

Ch'ng, Chin Lye. et al "Celiac Disease and Autoimmune Thyroid Disease." Clin Med Res. 2007 Oct; 5(3): 184–192

Spadaccino, AC, D. Basso, and S. Chiarelli. "Celiac Disease in North Italian Patients with Autoimmune Thyroid Diseases." Autoimmunity. 2008 Feb;41(1):116-21.

Kuma, Vijay, Jacobo Wortsman, and Manoj Rajadhyaksha. "Celiac Disease-Associated Autoimmune Endocrinopathies." Clin Diagn Lab Immunol. 2001 Jul; 8(4): 678–685

Collin, Pekka et al. "Autoimmune Thyroid Disorders and Coeliac Disease."*Eje-online.org.* European Society of Endocrinology.

MN, Akcay, G, Akcay "The Presence of the Antigliadin Antibodies in Autoimmune Thyroid Diseases."Hepatogastroenterology . 2003 Dec;50

Sategna-Guidetti, C et al. "Autoimmune Thyroid Diseases and Coeliac Disease." Clin Med Res. 2007 Oct; 5(3): 184–192
Yao, C. et al."Inhibitory Effects of Thyroxine on Cytokine Production by T Cells in Mice." Int Immunopharmacol. 2007 Dec 15;7(13):1747-54

Strieder, TG, MF Prummel, JG Tijssen, E. Endert, and WM Wiersinga. "Risk Factors for and Prevalence of Thyroid Disorders in a Cross-sectional Study among Healthy Female Relatives of Patients with Autoimmune Thyroid Disease." Clin Endocrinol (Oxf). 2003 Sep;59(3):396-401

Hakanen, M., K. Luotola, J. Salmi, P. Laippala , K. Kaukinen, and P. Collin."Clinical and Subclinical Autoimmune Thyroid Disease in Adult Celiac Disease." Dig Dis Sci 2001 Dec;46(12):2631-5

Kresser, Chris. "The Gluten-Thyroid Connection." ChrisKresser.com. Chris Kresser, 18 July 2010.

Denham, Jolanda M., and Ivor D. Hill. "Celiac Disease and Autoimmunity: Review and Controversies." Curr Allergy Asthma Rep. 2013; 13(4): 347–353

407

Hodkinson, Clare F. et al."Preliminary Evidence of Immune Function Modulation by Thyroid Hormones in Healthy Men and Women Aged 55–70 Years." Society for Endocrinology, 1 Apr. 2009.

Kumar, Vijay, Wortsman, Jacobo and RajadhyakshaManoj. "Celiac Disease-Associated Autoimmune Endocrinopathies." http://cvi.asm.org/. American Society for Microbiology.

Fasano, Alessio. "Systemic Autoimmune Disorders in Celiac Disease." Direct-ms.org. Lippincott Williams & Wilkins, 2006.

"Anti-transglutaminase Antibodies." En.wikipedia.org. Wikimedia Foundation.

Braunstein,Glenn.''The Effect of Celiac Disease on the Absorption of Levothyroxine Tablets.'' *Thyroid.org*. American Thyroid Association.

Caja, Sergio, Mäki, Markku, Kaukinen, Katri and Lindfors, Katri. "Antibodies in Celiac Disease: Implications beyond Diagnostics." Nature.com. Cellular & Molecular Immunology, 31 Jan. 2011.

Hadithi, Muhammed, De Boer, Hans, Meijer, Jos WR, Willekens, Franz, Kerckhaert, Jo A, Heijmans, Roel, Salvador Pena, Amado, Stehouwer, Coen DA, and Mulder, Chris JJ"Coeliac Disease in Dutch Patients with Hashimoto's Thyroiditis and Vice Versa." Wjgnet.com. World J Gastroenterol, 21 Mar. 2007.

Barton, Susan H., and, Murray, Joseph A. "Celiac Disease and Autoimmunity in the Gut and Elsewhere." Gastroenterol Clin North Am. 2008 Jun;37(2):411-vii.

Dach, Jeffrey. "Hashimotos Thyroid Disease and Molecular Mimicry." Http://jeffreydachmd.com/. Jeffrey Dach, 22 Jan. 2014.

Harris, Cheryl, and Kaplan, Gary. "Two of a Kind — Research Connects Celiac and Thyroid Diseases and Suggests a Gluten-Free Diet Benefits Both." Todaysdietitian.com. Great Valley Publishing Company, Inc, 1 Nov. 2010.

Kucera, P., Novakova, D., Behanova M, Novak J, Tlaskalova-Hogenova, H, and Andel M "Gliadin, Endomysial and Thyroid Antibodies in Patients with Latent Autoimmune Diabetes of Adults (LADA)." Clin Exp Immunol.. 2003 Jul;133(1):139-43

Fine, Kenneth. "Early Diagnosis Of Gluten Sensitivity: Before the Villi Are Gone." Enterolab.com. Specialized Laboratory Testing for Optimal Intestinal and Overall Health.

"Human Leukocyte Antigen." En.wikipedia.org. Wikimedia Foundation, Inc.

"Eating Gluten Increases the Need for Thyroid Hormones." Http://thyroidbook.com/. Datis Kharrazian, 19 Jan. 2012.

Martin, Antonio, De Vivo Giulia, and Gentile, Vittorio. "Possible Role of the Transglutaminases in the Pathogenesis of Alzheimer's Disease and Other Neurodegenerative Diseases." Hindawi.com. International Journal of Alzheimer's Disease.

Nakagawa, H., Fujii, A, Yoneda, M, Kinomoto, K, and Kuriyama, M. "Hashimoto's Encephalopathy Presenting with Progressive Cerebellar Ataxia." J Neurol Neurosurg Psychiatry. 2007 Feb; 78(2): 196–197

Hadjivassiliou, M., et al. "Gluten Ataxia in Perspective: Epidemiology, Genetic Susceptibility and Clinical Characteristics." Brain.2003 Mar;126(Pt 3):685-91

Seneff, Stephanie, and Samsel, Anthony. "Glyphosate, Pathways to Modern Diseases II: Celiac Sprue and Gluten Intolerance." Interdiscip Toxicol. 2013 Dec; 6(4): 159–184

Risk factors for and prevalence of thyroid disorders in a cross sectional study among healthy female relatives of patients with autoimmune thyroid disease. Clin Endocrinol (Oxf) 2003 Sep;59(3): 396-401

Julieta Gerenova, Manolova, Irena and Gadjeva, Veselina (2012). Hashimoto's Disease - Involvement of Cytokine Network and Role of Oxidative Stress in the Severity of Hashimoto's Thyroiditis, A New Look at Hypothyroidism, Dr. Drahomira Springer

409

Stress as a trigger of autoimmune disease Ljudmila Stojanovich □, Dragomir Marisavljevich "Bezhanijska Kosa" University Medical Center, Belgrade University, Serbia Autoimmunity, 2008 Feb;41(1):116=121

John R. Klein The Immune System as a Regulator of Thyroid Hormone Activity Exp Biol Med (Maywood). 2006 Mar; 231(3): 229–236.

Galland, Leo. "Leaky Gut Syndromes: Breaking the Vicious Cycle." Mdheal.org. Renaissance Workshops.Ltd.

"Candida Yeast Infection Leaky Gut, Irritable Bowel and Food Allergies." Nationalcandidacenter.com. National Candida Center.

Fratkin, Jake Paul. "Leaky Gut Syndrome: A Modern Epidemic Part I." Ei-resource.org. The Environmental Illness Resource, 1 Sept. 2014.

Brimberg L, Sadiq A, Gregersen PK, Diamond B. Brain-reactive IgG correlates with autoimmunity in mothers of a child with an autism spectrum disorder. Mol Psychiatry. 2013 Nov;18(11):1171-7. doi: 10.1038/mp.2013.101. Epub 2013 Aug 20.

Sapone, Anna.et al. "Spectrum of Gluten-related Disorders: Consensus on New Nomenclature and Classification." BMC Med. 2012; 10: 13

Trescott, Mickey. "How Do You Balance TH1 and TH2 in Autoimmune Disease?"autoimmune-paleo.com. Mickey Trescott, 24 Jan. 2013.

Ni, Maoshing. The Yellow Emperor's Classic of Medicine. Boston: Shambhala Publications, 1995.

Kharrazian, Datis. "Autoimmune Thyroid" *Mastering the Thyroid*. Datis Kharrazian, 2011. 251

Pitchford, Paul. "Metal Element." *Healing with Whole Foods: Oriental Traditions and Modern Nutrition.* Revised ed. Berkeley: North Atlantic, 1993. 306-314.

Liu, Master Hong. The Healing Art of Qi Gong Healing. New York: Warner, 1997.

Chapter 10-12: (Earth Element)

Email from Dr. Izabella Wentz entitled: "Top 10 Takeaways from 2232 People with Hashimoto's" received June 21st, 2015. Survey conducted in May of 2015.

Here are some additional findings from this email:

"1) Stress is a huge contributing factor! 69% of you reported that you had a lot of stress in your life before you started feeling unwell.

2) Nutrient deficiencies are real! 68%, 33% and 28% of you were found to have low levels of Vitamin D, low levels of B12 and low levels of ferritin, respectively.

Taking supplements can help restore your nutrient levels and help overcome fatigue. When asked about the benefits of various interventions, 67%, 88%, 82%, reported that Vitamin D3, B12 and Iron/ferritin supplements improved their fatigue, respectively.

3) Gluten sensitivity with Hashimoto's is a big deal. 76% of you reported that you thought you were gluten sensitive (16% of you were not sure, the rest did not believe that you were)…

…Overall, 88% of people who attempted to go gluten-free felt better!! 86% of people who went gluten-free reported an improvement in digestive symptoms.

Notably, only 3.5% of you were actually diagnosed with celiac disease, thus this confirms what we've been saying all along, you do not have to have celiac disease to benefit from a gluten-free diet!

4) Food matters! In addition to the gluten-free diet, the other most helpful dietary interventions were going on a sugar free diet and the Paleo diet (81% of those who tried these diets felt better), grain-free diet (81% felt better), dairy free diet (79% felt better), autoimmune Paleo diet (75% felt better) and the low glycemic index diet (76% felt better). Incorporating healing foods also made people feel better. Home-made broth helped 70% of those that tried it, Green smoothies helped 69%, and fermented foods helped 57%.

5) Supplements can help. The most helpful nutritional interventions were taking a B12 supplement(76%), D3 supplement (74%), digestive enzymes (73%), Ferritin/Iron supplement (63%), Omega-3 Fatty acid supplement (65%), Selenium 200 mcg (63%), Betaine with Pepsin (59%), Curcumin (56%),Zinc 30 mg (52%) and L-glutamine (51%). (The numbers in the parentheses represent the % of people who reported "feeling better" after trying these supplements).

6) Sauna therapy helped an overall 57% of those who tried it to feel better, the biggest benefits were seen in mood, energy, skin and reducing pain levels. Massage helped improve mood for 80% of people, reduced pain for 62% and improved energy levels in 45% of people! …

8) Sweet spot for TSH levels. 69% of respondents feel optimal with a TSH under 1 μIU/ml, and 57% felt good with the TSH between 1 and 2 μIU/ml !! While a TSH as high as 4 μIU/ml may be considered to be "within normal limits" I personally felt like a sloth and was losing a ton of hair when my TSH was at that level…

10)Probiotics can help normalize weight- 36% of people felt that probiotics helped them normalize their weight. "

Maclean, Will, Lyttleton, Jane. Clinical Handbook of Internal Medicine: The Treatment of Disease with Traditional Chinese Medicine. Vol. 2: Spleen and Stomach: Chinese Medicine Unit of the Faculty Health, U of Western Sydney Macarthur, 2002.

Drossman, Douglas. "Brain-gut Connections in Functional GI Disorders: Anatomic and Physiologic Relationships." *Researchgate.net.* Blackwell, 1 Mar. 2006.

Guinane,Caitriona M, et al. "Microbial Composition of Human Appendices from Patients following Appendectomy." Http://mbio.asm.org/. American Society for Microbiology.

Sachmechi, I., DM Reich, and M. Aninyei.etc "Effect of Proton Pump Inhibitors on Serum Thyroid-stimulating Hormone Level in Euthyroid Patients Treated with Levothyroxine for Hypothyroidism." Endocr Pract 2007 Jul-Aug;13(4):345-9

Chen, John K., and Tina T. Chen. Chinese Medical Herbology and Pharmacology. Industry: Art of Medicine, 2001.

Kendall, Donald E. Dao of Chinese Medicine: Understanding an Ancient Healing Art. Oxford: Oxford UP, 2002.

Jarrett, Lonny S. "Earth-The Axis." Nourishing Destiny: The Inner Tradition of Chinese Medicine. Stockbridge: Spirit Path, 1998. 278-298.

Kharrazian, Datis. Mastering the Thyroid. Datis Kharrazian, 2011.

Kharrazian, Datis. Why Do I Still Have Thyroid Symptoms?:When My Lab Tests Are Normal. Carlsbad: Elephant Printing, LLC, 2010.

Benschoten, Van. Autoimmune Disease and Chinese Herbal Medicine. Santa Monica: Emperor's College of Oriental Medicine, 2003

Autoimmune Disease, Multiple Chemical Disorders, and Chinese Medicine, M.M. Van Benchotten, O.M.D., Lotus Institute of integrative Medicine, 2009

Braverman, Lewis E., and Robert D. Utiger. "Section C. Organ System Manifestations of Hypothyroidism." Werner & Ingbar's-The Thyroid: A Fundamental and Clinical Text. 9th ed. Philadelphia: Lippincott Williams & Wilkins, 2005. 796-802.

Kresser, Chris. "The Hidden Causes of Heartburn and GERD." Chriskresser.com. Chris Kresser, 1 Apr. 2010.

Harvey, Sugerman. "Increased Intra-abdominal Pressure and GERD/Barrett's Esophagus." Gastrojournal.org. Elsevier, 4 Mar. 2014.

Theisen, Jörg, et al."Suppression of Gastric Acid Secretion in Patients with Gastroesophageal Reflux Disease Results in Gastric Bacterial Overgrowth and Deconjugation of Bile Acids." Link.springer.com. Journal of Gastrointestinal Surgery, 2000.

Kresser, Chris. "Thyroid, Blood Sugar, and Metabolic Syndrome." Chriskresser.com. Chris Kresser, 23 July 2010.

R, Kadiyala, R, Peter, and OE, Okosieme. "Thyroid Dysfunction in Patients with Diabetes: Clinical Implications and Screening Strategies."Int J Clin Pract. 2010 Jul;64(8):1130-9

J, Ahmad, F, Ahmed , and MA, Siddiqui. "Inflammation, Insulin Resistance and Carotid IMT in First Degree Relatives of North Indian Type 2 Diabetic Subjects.". Diabetes Res Clin Pract.2006 Aug;73(2):205-10

Kresser, Chris. "The Thyroid-Gut Connection." Chriskresser.com. Chris Kresser, 9 July 2010.

Stratakis, CA, and GP Chrousos. "Neuroendocrinology and Pathophysiology of the Stress System." Ann NY Acad Sci. 1995 Dec 29;771:1-18

Van Der Poll, T, et al. "Interleukin-1 Receptor Blockade Does Not Affect Endotoxin-induced Changes in Plasma Thyroid Hormone and Thyrotropin Concentrations in Man." J Clin Endocrinol Metab 1995 Apr;80(4):1341-6

Mandrup-Poulsen, Thomas, et al. "Cytokines and the Endocrine System. II. Roles in Substrate Metabolism, Modulation of Thyroidal and Pancreatic Endocrine Cell Functions and Autoimmune Endocrine Diseases." Eje-online.org. European Society of Endocrinology.

Singleton, J. Robinson, Smith, Gordon A., and Bromberg, Mark B.,. "Increased Prevalence of Impaired Glucose Tolerance in Patients With Painful Sensory Neuropathy." Care.diabetesjournals.org. American Diabetes Association.

Holtorf, Kent. "Insulin Resistance Can Trigger Hashimoto's Disease." Nahypothyroidism.org. National Academy of Hypothyroidism, 10 Apr. 2013.

Nichols, Gregory A, Hillier, Teresa A., and Brown, Jonathan B.,. "Normal Fasting Plasma Glucose and Risk of Type 2 Diabetes Diagnosis." Amjmed.com. Elsevier Inc, 1 June 2008.

Tirosh, A., et al. "Normal Fasting Plasma Glucose Levels and Type 2 Diabetes in Young Men." N Engl J Med.2005 Oct 6;353(14):1454-62

Donahue R, Abbott R, Reed D, Yano K. Postchallenge glucose concentration and coronary heart disease in men of Japanese ancestry. Honolulu Heart Program. Diabetes. 1987;36(6):689–692.

Lowe L, Liu K, Greenland P, Metzger B, Dyer A, Stamler J. Diabetes, asymptomatic hyperglycemia, and 22-year mortality in black and white men. The Chicago Heart Association Detection Project in Industry Study. Diabetes Care. 1997;20(2):163–169.

Balkau B, Shipley M, Jarrett R, Pyörälä K, Pyörälä M, Forhan A, Eschwège E. High blood glucose concentration is a risk factor for mortality in middle-aged nondiabetic men. 20-year follow-up in the Whitehall Study, the Paris Prospective Study, and the Helsinki Policemen Study. Diabetes Care. 1998;21(3):360–367.

De Vegt F, Dekker JM, Ruhè HG, Stehouwer CD, Nijpels G, Bouter LM, Heine RJ. Hyperglycaemia is associated with all-cause and cardiovascular mortality in the Hoorn population: the Hoorn Study. Diabetologia.1999;42(8):926–931.

Esposito K, Ciotola M, Carleo D, Schisano B, Sardelli L, Di Tommaso D, Misso L, Saccomanno F, Ceriello A, Giugliano D. Post-meal glucose peaks at home associate with carotid intima-media thickness in type 2 diabetes.J Clin Endocrinol Metab. 2008;93(4):1345–1350.

Lenzen, S., HG Joost, and A. Hasselblatt. "Thyroid Function and Insulin Secretion from the Perfused Pancreas in the Rat." Endocrinology 1976 Jul;99(1):125-9

Gullo, L., et al. "Influence of the Thyroid on Exocrine Pancreatic Function.". Gastroenterology. 1991 May;100(5 Pt 1):1392-6

Malaisse, Willy J, Francine Malaisse-Lagae, and Edward F McCraw. "Effects of Thyroid Function upon Insulin Secretion."diabetes.diabetesjournals.org. 1 Sept. 1967. 16:9 643-646

Potenza, M., MA Via, and RT Yanagisawa. "Excess Thyroid Hormone and Carbohydrate Metabolism." Endocr Pract. 2009 Apr;15(3):254-62.

Campbell, T. Colin. "Low Fat Diets Are Grossly Misrepresented." Huffingtonpost.com. Thehuffingtonpost.com, Inc, 17 Nov. 2011.

Galland, Leo. "Leaky Gut Syndromes: Breaking the Vicious Cycle." Mdheal.org. Renaissance Workshops.Ltd.

"Candida Yeast Infection Leaky Gut, Irritable Bowel and Food Allergies." Nationalcandidacenter.com. National Candida Center.

Fratkin, Jake Paul. "Leaky Gut Syndrome: A Modern Epidemic Part II." Ei-resource.org. The Environmental Illness Resource, 1 Sept. 2014.

Arrieta, M C et al. "Alterations in Intestinal Permeability." Gut. 2006 Oct; 55(10): 1512–1520

Reardon, Sara. "Gut–brain Link Grabs Neuroscientists." Nature.com. Nature Publishing Group, 14 Nov. 2014.

"The Brain-Gut Connection." Hopkinsmedicine.org. The Johns Hopkins University, The Johns Hopkins Hospital, and Johns Hopkins Health System.

Granito, A., et al. "Anti-actin IgA Antibodies in Severe Coeliac Disease."
Clin Exp Immunol. 2004 Aug; 137(2): 386–392

Vogelsang H, Wyatt J, Penner E, Lochs H. Screening for celiac disease in first-degree relatives of patients with celiac disease by lactulose/mannitol test. Am J Gastroenterol. 1995 Oct;90(10):1838-42.

Molodecky, Natalie A., and Kaplan, Gilaad G. "Environmental Risk Factors for Inflammatory Bowel Disease." Gastroenterol Hepatol (N Y). 2010 May; 6(5): 339–346

"Array 2- Antibody: Intestinal Antigenic Permeability Screen." Clinical Application Guide (2011).

Blaser MJ (2006). "Who are we? Indigenous microbes and the ecology of human diseases" (PDF). EMBO Reports 7 (10): 956–60.doi:10.1038 /sj.embor.7400812. PMC 1618379. PMID 17016449.

Kharrazian, Datis. Why Do I Still Have Thyroid Symptoms?:When My Lab Tests Are Normal. Carlsbad: Elephant Printing, LLC, 2010.

Kendall, Donald E. Dao of Chinese Medicine: Understanding an Ancient Healing Art. Oxford: Oxford UP, 2002.

Pitchford, Paul. "Earth Element." Healing with Whole Foods: Oriental Traditions and Modern Nutrition. Revised ed. Berkeley: North Atlantic, 1993. 302-306, 334.

Ni, Maoshing. The Yellow Emperor's Classic of Medicine. Boston: Shambhala Publications, 1995.

Trescott, Mickey. The Autoimmune Paleo Cookbook. Mickey Trescott, 2014.

Liu, Master Hong. The Healing Art of Qi Gong Healing. New York: Warner, 1997.

Chapter 13-17: (Water Element)

Agmon-Levin, N. et al. "Vitamin D in Systemic and Organ-specific Autoimmune Diseases." 2013 Oct;45(2):256-66

"9 Things That Can Undermine Your Vitamin D Level." *Health.harvard.edu*. Harvard Health.

Tzu, Lao, and John C. H. Wu. *Tao Te Ching*. Boston: Shambhala Publications, 1961. Print.

Klein, Irwin, Danzi, Sarah. "Cardiovascular Involvement in General Medical Conditions: Thyroid Disease and the Heart." American Heart Association.

Kendall, Donald E. Dao of Chinese Medicine: Understanding an Ancient Healing Art. Oxford: Oxford UP, 2002.

Jarrett, Lonny S. "Water-The Great." Nourishing Destiny: The Inner Tradition of Chinese Medicine. Stockbridge: Spirit Path, 1998. 176-198.

Braverman, Lewis E., and Robert D. Utiger. "Section C. Organ System Manifestations of Hypothyroidism-." Werner & Ingbar's-The Thyroid: A Fundamental and Clinical Text. 9th ed. Philadelphia: Lippincott Williams & Wilkins, 2005. 789-795, 811-816.

Kharrazian, Datis. Why Do I Still Have Thyroid Symptoms?:When My Lab Tests Are Normal. Carlsbad: Elephant Printing, LLC, 2010.

Pitchford, Paul. "Water Element." *Healing with Whole Foods: Oriental Traditions and Modern Nutrition*. Revised ed. Berkeley: North Atlantic, 1993. 315-328.

Chen, John K., and Tina T. Chen. *Chinese Medical Herbology and Pharmacology*. Industry: Art of Medicine, 2001.

"Understanding the Adrenal and Thyroid Connection." Holtorfmed.com. Holtorf Medical Group.

Kresser, Chris. "5 Ways That Stress Causes Hypothyroid Symptoms." Chriskresser.com. Chris Kresser, 10 Aug. 2010.

BioHealth Diagnoistics "Understanding Adrenal Function." Http://articles.mercola.com/. Dr. Joseph Mercola, 1 Aug.27. 2000.

Kresser, Chris. "The Role of Vitamin D Deficiency in Thyroid Disorders." Chriskresser.com. Chris Kresser, 4 Aug. 2010.

"Metabolic Temperature Graph." Drrind.com. Dr. Rind.

McCann, SM, Jurcovicova, J and V. Rettori. "Central Action of Interleukin-1 in Altering the Release of TSH, Growth Hormone, and Prolactin in the Male Rat." J Neurosci Res. 1987;18(1):179-83

XP, Pang, et al. "Impairment of Hypothalamic-pituitary-thyroid Function in Rats Treated with Human Recombinant Tumor Necrosis Factor-alpha (cachectin)." Endocrinology. 1989 Jul;125(1):76-84

P, Caturegli, , Kimura, H. "Chemokine Orchestration of Autoimmune Thyroiditis." Thyroid.2007 Oct;17(10):1005-11

F, Baeke et al."Vitamin D: Modulator of the Immune System." 1 Aug. 2010.

Kharrazian, Datis. Mastering the Thyroid. Datis Kharrazian, 2011.

Ni, Maoshing. The Yellow Emperor's Classic of Medicine. Boston: Shambhala Publications, 1995.

Liu, Master Hong. The Healing Art of Qi Gong Healing. New York: Warner, 1997.

Chapter 18-20: (The Brain)

Pert, Candace. Molecules of Emotion: Why You Feel the Way You Feel. Scribner.

Davidison, Richard J. The Emotional Life of Your Brain: How It's Unique Patterns Affect the Way You Think, Feel, and Live -and How You Can Change Them. Hudson Street, 2012.

Mallat, M., et al. "New Insights into the Role of Thyroid Hormone in the CNS: The Microglial Track." Nature.com.

Lima, Flavia R.S. et al. "Regulation of Microglial Development: A Novel Role for Thyroid Hormone." Jneurosci.org. The Journal of Neuroscience, 15 Mar. 2001.

De La Monte, Suzanne M. et al. "Alzheimer's Disease Is Type 3 Diabetes–Evidence Reviewed." J Diabetes Sci Technol. 2008 Nov; 2(6): 1101–1113

Kharrazzian, Datis. "Thyroid-Brain Crosstalk-Part 1: The Microglia, Neuron and Thyroid Connection." Http://sanjosefuncmed.com/. San Jose Functional Medicine, 12 Nov. 2010.

Harry, G. Jean, and Kraft, Andrew D "Microglia in the Developing Brain: A Potential Target with Lifetime Effects." Ff.ul.pt.

Bonuccelli, U., et al "Thyroid Function and Autoimmunity in Parkinson's Disease: A Study of 101 Patients."Parkinsonism Relat Disord. 1999 Apr;5(1-2):49-53

Huang, MJ. et al. "Clinical Associations between Thyroid and Liver Diseases."J Gastroenterol Hepatol. 1995 May-Jun;10(3):344-50

Bowem, R. "Thyroid Hormones: Pregnancy and Fetal Development." Vivo.colostate.edu. 26 Feb. 2012.

Escobar G, De Morreale. "The Role of Thyroid Hormone in Fetal Neurodevelopment." J Pediatr endocrinol Metab. 2001;14 Suppl 6:1453-62

Patel, J., et al. "Thyroid Hormones and Fetal Neurological Development.". J Endocrinol. 2011 Apr;209(1):1-8

Houston Methodist. "Autism four times likelier when mother's thyroid is weakened." ScienceDaily. ScienceDaily, 13 August 2013.

Mittelbronn, Michel, et al. "CD8 /perforin /granzyme B Effector Cells Infiltrating Cerebellum and Inferior Olives in Gluten Ataxia." Http://onlinelibrary.wiley.com/. Japanese Society of Neuropathology.

Zoeller, Thomas R, et al. "Thyroid Hormone, Brain Development, and the Environment." Environ Health Perspect. 2002 Jun; 110(Suppl 3): 355–361

Trentini, Dana. "Maternal Hypothyroidism And Fetal Brain Development." Hypothyroidmom.com. Prose Theme on Genesis Framework, 13 May 2013.

Bernal, Juan. "Thyroid Hormones in Brain Development and Function." Thyroidmanager.org. Thyroid Disease Manager, 17 Dec. 2012.

Ganguli M, Burmeister LA, Seaberg EC, Belle S, DeKosky ST. Association between dementia and elevated TSH: a community-based study. Biol. Psychiatr. 1996; 40: 714-725.

Schiess, N., and CA Pardo. "Hashimoto's Encephalopathy." Ann NY Acad Sci. 2008 Oct;1142:254-65

Wang, Jianhong, et al "Cognitive Impairments in Hashimoto's Encephalopathy: A Case-Control Study." Http://journals.plos.org/. 8 Feb. 2013.

Selim, M, and Drachman, D. "Ataxia Associated with Hashimoto's Disease: Progressive Non-familial Adult Onset Cerebellar Degeneration with Autoimmune Thyroiditis." J Neurol Neurosurg Psychiatry. 2001 Jul; 71(1): 81–87

"The Effects of Hashimoto's and Hypothyroidism on Brain Health." Http://drknews.com/. Datis Kharrazian, 17 Feb. 2010.

Braverman, Lewis E., and Robert D. Utiger. "Section C. Organ System Manifestations of Hypothyroidism." Werner & Ingbar's-The Thyroid: A Fundamental and Clinical Text. 9th ed. Philadelphia: Lippincott Williams & Wilkins, 2005. 836-850.

Kharrazian, Datis. Why Do I Still Have Thyroid Symptoms?:When My Lab Tests Are Normal. Carlsbad: Elephant Printing, LLC, 2010.

Wentz, Izabella. Hashimoto's Thyroiditis: Lifestyle Interventions for Finding and Treating the Root Cause. Izabella Wentz, PharmD, 2013.

"How Adrenals Can Wreak Havoc." Stopthethyroidmadness.com. Stop the Thyroid Madness.

Lam, Michael. "The Adrenal Glands." Tuberrose.com.

"Dietary Sources of Omega-3 Fatty Acids." *Dietary Sources of Omega-3 Fatty Acids*.

Chapter 21-24: (The Wood Element)

Rigopoulou, Eirini I. et al "Epstein-Barr Virus as a Trigger of Autoimmune Liver Diseases." 2012.

Oliva, Francesco. "Thyroid Hormones and Tendon: Current Views and Future Perspectives. Concise Review." Muscles Ligaments Tendons J. 2013 Jul-Sep; 3(3): 201–203

Pitchford, Paul. "Wood Element." *Healing with Whole Foods: Oriental Traditions and Modern Nutrition*. Revised ed. Berkeley: North Atlantic, 1993. 84-290.

Murrell, G A. "Understanding Tendinopathies." BJ Sports Med, 2002;36:392–393

Beinfield, Harriet, and Efrem Korngold. Between Heaven and Earth. Ballantine, 1991.

Bensky, Dan, Barolet, Randall. Chinese Herbal Medicine Formulas and Strategies. Seattle: Eastland, 1990.

Kendall, Donald E. Dao of Chinese Medicine: Understanding an Ancient Healing Art. Oxford: Oxford UP, 2002.

Jarrett, Lonny S. "Wood-Far Away" Nourishing Destiny: The Inner Tradition of Chinese Medicine. Stockbridge: Spirit Path, 1998. 234-256.

Braverman, Lewis E., and Robert D. Utiger. "Section C. Organ System Manifestations of Hypothyroidism." Werner & Ingbar's-The Thyroid: A Fundamental and Clinical Text. 9th ed. Philadelphia: Lippincott Williams & Wilkins, 2005. 796-802.

Kharrazian, Datis. Why Do I Still Have Thyroid Symptoms?:When My Lab Tests Are Normal. Carlsbad: Elephant Printing, LLC, 2010.

Wentz, Izabella. Hashimoto's Thyroiditis: Lifestyle Interventions for Finding and Treating the Root Cause. Izabella Wentz, PharmD, 2013.

Ni, Maoshing. The Yellow Emperor's Classic of Medicine. Boston: Shambhala Publications, 1995.

Severe hyperthyroidism induces mitochondria-mediated apoptosis in rat liver. Upadhyay G, Singh R, Kumar A, Kumar S, Kapoor A, Godbole MM. Source:Department of Endocrinology, Sanjay Gandhi Postgraduate Institute of Medical Sciences, Lucknow, India.

Laukkarinen J, Kiudelis G, Lempinen M, Raty S, Pelli H, Sand J, Kemppainen E, Haglund C, Nordback I. Increased prevalence of subclinical hypothyroidism in common bile duct stone patients. J Clin Endocrinol Metab. 2007 Nov;92(11):4260-4. Epub 2007 Aug 28

Inkinen J, Sand J, Nordback I. Association between common bile duct stones and treated hypothyroidism. Hepatogastroenterology. 2000 Jul-Aug:47(34):919-21

Liu, Master Hong. The Healing Art of Qi Gong Healing. New York: Warner, 1997.

Chapter 25-29: (The Fire Element)

Maclean, Will, and Jane Lyttleton. Clinical Handbook of Internal Medicine: The Treatment of Disease with Traditional Chinese Medicine. Vol. 1: Lung, Kidney, Liver, and Heart. Campbeltown: Chinese Medicine Unit of the Faculty Health, U of Western Sydney Macarthur, 1998.

Chen, John K., Chen, Tina T. Chinese Medical Herbology and Pharmacology. Industry: Art of Medicine, 2001.

Kendall, Donald E. Dao of Chinese Medicine: Understanding an Ancient Healing Art. Oxford: Oxford UP, 2002.

Jarrett, Lonny S. "Fire-Moving Away." Nourishing Destiny: The Inner Tradition of Chinese Medicine. Stockbridge: Spirit Path, 1998. 196-232.

Braverman, Lewis E., and Robert D. Utiger. "Section C. Organ System Manifestations of Hypothyroidism." Werner & Ingbar's-The Thyroid: A Fundamental and Clinical Text. 9th ed. Philadelphia: Lippincott Williams & Wilkins, 2005. 774-781, 790.

Kharrazian, Datis. Why Do I Still Have Thyroid Symptoms?:When My Lab Tests Are Normal. Carlsbad: Elephant Printing, LLC, 2010.

Kendall, Donald E. Dao of Chinese Medicine: Understanding an Ancient Healing Art. Oxford: Oxford UP, 2002.

Jarrett, Lonny S. "Metal-The Return." Nourishing Destiny: The Inner Tradition of Chinese Medicine. Stockbridge: Spirit Path, 1998. 258-276.

Ni, Maoshing. The Yellow Emperor's Classic of Medicine. Boston: Shambhala Publications, 1995.

Pitchford, Paul. "Fire Element." *Healing with Whole Foods: Oriental Traditions and Modern Nutrition*. Revised ed. Berkeley: North Atlantic, 1993. 296-299.

Lauritano, EC, et al. "Association between Hypothyroidism and Small Intestinal Bacterial Overgrowth."J Clin Endocrinol Metab. 2007 Nov;92(11):4180-4

Tursi, A., Brandimarte. G, and Giorgetti, G. "High Prevalence of Small Intestinal Bacterial Overgrowth in Celiac Patients with Persistence of Gastrointestinal Symptoms after Gluten Withdrawal." Am J Gastroenterol. 2003 Apr;98(4):839-43

Wolfson, Allan B et al. *Harwood-Nuss' Clinical Practice of Emergency Medicine*. 5th ed. Philadelphia: Lippincott Williams & Wilkins, 2010.

Fasano, A. "Leaky Gut and Autoimmune Diseases."Clin Rev Allergy Immunol. 2012 Feb;42(1):71-8

Fazio, Serafino et al. "Effects of Thyroid Hormone on the Cardiovascular System."

Klein, Irwin, and Kaie Ojamaa. "Thyroid Hormone and the Cardiovascular System." Massachusetts Medical Society, 2001;344:501-509

Urita, Y., et al. "Extensive Atrophic Gastritis Increases Intraduodenal Hydrogen Gas." Gastroenterol Res Pract. 2008; 2008

Axon, A., and G, Naylor, "Role of Bacterial Overgrowth in the Stomach as an Additional Risk Factor for Gastritis." Can J Gastroenterol..2003 Jun;17

Soifer, LO. et al "[Comparative Clinical Efficacy of a Probiotic vs. an Antibiotic in the Treatment of Patients with Intestinal Bacterial Overgrowth and Chronic Abdominal Functional Distension: A Pilot Study]."Acta Gastroenterol Latinoam. 2010 Dec;40(4):323-7

Henriksson, et al. "Small Intestinal Bacterial Overgrowth in Patients with Rheumatoid Arthritis." Ann Rheum Dis. 1993 Jul; 52(7): 503–510

"Blood Pressure Problems and Hypothyroidism Can Go Hand-in-hand." Stopthethyroidmadness.com. Stop the Thyroid Madness.

Davis, PJ Et Al. "Interaction of Thyroid Hormone and Hemoglobin. I. Nature of the Interaction and Effect of Hemoglobin on Thyroid Hormone Radioimmunoassay."J Lab Clin Med. 1980 May;95(5):714-24

Bures, J. "Modifying Paleo for Small Intestinal Bacterial Overgrowth." Thepaleomom.com. World J Gastroenterol, 1 June 2010.

Liu, Master Hong. The Healing Art of Qi Gong Healing. New York: Warner, 1997.